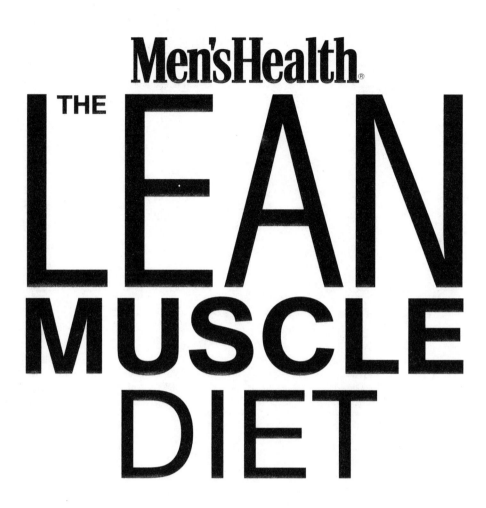

Men'sHealth ®

THE

LEAN

MUSCLE

DIET

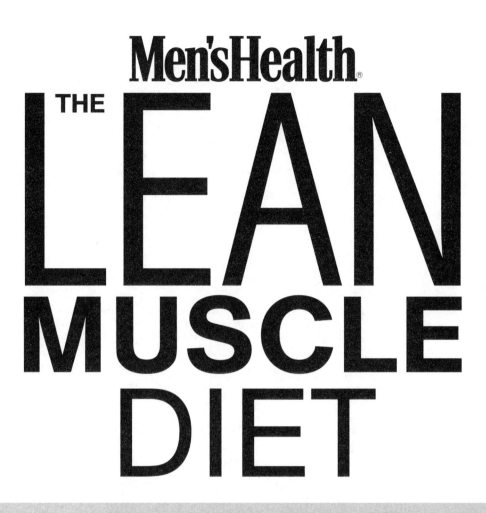

Men'sHealth®
THE LEAN MUSCLE DIET

A CUSTOMIZED NUTRITION AND WORKOUT PLAN— EAT THE FOODS YOU LOVE TO BUILD THE BODY YOU WANT AND KEEP IT FOR LIFE!

LOU SCHULER AND **ALAN ARAGON,** MS

RODALE.

NOTICE

The information in this book is meant to supplement, not replace, proper exercise training. All forms of exercise pose some inherent risks. The editors and publisher advise readers to take full responsibility for their safety and know their limits. Before practicing the exercises in this book, be sure that your equipment is well-maintained, and do not take risks beyond your level of experience, aptitude, training, and fitness. The exercise and dietary programs in this book are not intended as a substitute for any exercise routine or dietary regimen that may have been prescribed by your doctor. As with all exercise and dietary programs, you should get your doctor's approval before beginning.

Mention of specific companies, organizations, or authorities in this book does not imply endorsement by the author or publisher, nor does mention of specific companies, organizations, or authorities imply that they endorse this book, its author, or the publisher.

Internet addresses and telephone numbers given in this book were accurate at the time it went to press.

Rodale books may be purchased for business or promotional use or for special sales. For information, please write to: Special Markets Department, Rodale, Inc., 733 Third Avenue, New York, NY 10017

Men'sHealth is a registered trademark of Rodale Inc.

Printed in the United States of America

Rodale Inc. makes every effort to use acid-free ∞, recycled paper ♻.

Photographs by Tom MacDonald

Book design by Elizabeth Neal

Library of Congress Cataloging-in-Publication Data is on file with the publisher.

ISBN 978-1-62336-418-2 hardcover

Distributed to the trade by Macmillan

2 4 6 8 10 9 7 5 3 1 hardcover

We inspire and enable people to improve their lives and the world around them.
rodalebooks.com

CONTENTS:

ACKNOWLEDGMENTS:

The longer I do this, the more indebted I feel to the many individuals who help me. I struggled to stay awake in my science classes in high school and college, which means I depend on a network of fitness and nutrition professionals to help me understand the complexities of their fields. Few have been more generous with their time and expertise than my coauthor, Alan Aragon. For as long as I've known him, he's been a valuable source of both strong opinions and data to back them up.

Same goes for all the experts who answer my emails with patience and good humor, including past and future coauthors Alwyn Cosgrove and Chad Waterbury. Thanks very much to Bret Contreras, Brad Schoenfeld, Mike T. Nelson, Dr. Spencer Nadolsky, Eric Cressey, Mike Roussell, Dean Somerset, Jon Fass, Nick Tumminello, and probably dozens more. And I owe much more than thanks to Dr. Bryan Chung, a research methodologist who helps me interpret studies that would otherwise be incomprehensible. One time when I was past deadline he answered my questions in between sets of his own workout.

None of their knowledge would reach our readers if not for my friends and colleagues at *Men's Health* and Rodale Books, including Jeff Csatari, Mike Zimmerman, Adam Campbell, Bill Phillips, and Peter Moore; Gregg Stebben of Men's Health Radio; photographer Tom MacDonald; model Thomas Canestraro; and designer Elizabeth Neal. And big thanks, as always, to David Black and Sarah Smith of the David Black Agency.

I'm also indebted, for many reasons, to Nick Bromberg, Sol Orwell, Dick Talens, Jon Goodman, Jean-Paul Francoeur, Roland Denzel, Dave Tropeano, Chris Leavy, and John Graham and Brian Zarbatany at St. Luke's Sports and Human Performance Center.

I'm eternally grateful to Kimberly Heinrichs, my long-suffering wife, and Harrison, Meredith, and Annie, our intermittently suffering kids. But the biggest thanks of all go to the readers who've supported my work so generously and enthusiastically for so many years. You never fail to challenge, motivate, and inspire me.

—L.S.

I would first like to thank Lou Schuler for seeing the merit of my work and giving me the opportunity to collaborate with him. I first became aware of him through the ubiquitous raves over *The New Rules of Lifting*, and have admired his work ever since. Fast-forward nearly a decade later, and here we are joining forces on a book that I could not be happier with.

I owe tremendous gratitude to my incredible wife Jeana and my wonderful sons Lex and Max—your patience and love have been immeasurable. It goes without saying that the support of everyone in my immediate and extended family has been foundational for me in all aspects.

I am indebted to Lyle McDonald for encouraging my plunge into the fierce and fascinating world of science-based information, and to Brad Schoenfeld for his sage guidance and partnership in conducting the very research comprising our scientific knowledge. I would also like to thank Eric Helms, Peter Fitschen, and James Krieger for their co-authorship in our contributions to the peer-reviewed literature.

Adam Campbell and Adam Bornstein have a special place on my thank-you list for strong-arming me onto the Men's Health team. Thanks to all of the tireless staff at *Men's Health* who cast their votes of confidence and made this book a reality.

Last but not least, a huge thanks goes out to everyone who has followed my work since the beginning, as well as those who just started. You make my career the deeply gratifying and meaningful adventure that it is.

—*A.A.*

BECAUSE IT'S HARD

s I write this, there are just over 7 billion people on the planet. The majority of them are too busy with daily life to obsess over how they look with their clothes off. But that still leaves a few hundred million—including every single person reading this page—who worry about their appearance, and who are willing to do something to improve it. The open question is the best way to accomplish that goal.

This should be straightforward. You need to know just three things.

▶ **Where you are now.** Measure anything that matters to you, and that you can manipulate with some combination of diet, exercise, and behavior. Weight, waist size, and upper-arm girth are malleable. Height and hair follicle density aren't.

▶ **Where you want to be.** Trickier, right? It's easy enough to say, "I want to lose 15 pounds." But 15 pounds of what? What do you want to look like after you reach your goal? I don't know you personally, but it's hard to believe you want to look exactly the same—a narrower version of your flabby-ass self, or a thicker version of the stick-figure guy you see in the mirror—and your only concern is a number on your bathroom scale. You don't want to settle for "smaller" or "bigger." You want to look better.

▶ **How to get there.** If you knew how to do this, you probably wouldn't be reading this book in the first place. Chances are good it's not your first attempt to change the way your body looks. Nor, for that matter, is it the first time I've written a book about how to change it. So why hasn't it worked for you?

Throughout this book, my coauthor and I will describe dozens of problems, solutions, and problems with the potential solutions. We'll give the best guidance possible on what to do and what to avoid, and explain in sometimes painful detail why the practices we recommend work better than others for most people who try them. But right now, in just three words, I'll tell you the single biggest reason why so many of us struggle to lose fat, build muscle, and change our appearance in a satisfying way.

Because it's hard.

More important are these five words: *It's supposed to be hard.* A mature human body is built for homeostasis. It wants to stay the same.

Consider this: A hungry guy might put away a million calories in a year. The daily average would be 2,750 calories, but nobody eats the exact same amount of food every day. The number will probably fluctuate by a couple hundred calories a day, with a little more on weekends and holidays and a little less on weekdays. And yet, the average American gains less than a pound over the course of a year. Think about that: a million calories, spread over 365 days, and by the end of the year your body has probably stored just 2,000 of them. Your body is *really good* at keeping you in balance. The size and shape you are now is the exact size and shape you've conditioned your body to maintain.

There are no easy ways to make noticeable, measurable, bucket-list improvements in the way your body looks and performs. But of course you know this. You're too smart to believe the ads you see on your favorite Web sites, the ones with Photoshopped pictures of "this guy" who has "one weird trick" to make it all better. There's no "superfood" that turns fat into muscle. Nor is there any single food that destroys your metabolism, or anything else you can stop eating or doing to make all your problems go away.

If any of this were simple and easy, we'd all be magnificent human specimens, with lean, muscular bodies and abs we could rent out to a marching band in need of a glockenspiel. How many people do you know who look like that? Two, right? (That guy on YouTube doesn't count. You don't actually know him.) And chances are, if you ask one of those guys how he did it and how he continues to do it, you'll get a fantastically complicated answer. Ask both guys, and you'll get two fantastically complicated answers, with bonus points for contradicting each other.

But here's the question that matters most: How can you get into the best shape for *you*? That question is complicated, but not fantastically so. And really, it's more like three questions.

How do I lose fat?

How do I put on muscle?

How do I maintain a healthy weight and a great physique for the rest of my life?

All of those goals are attainable. With *The Lean Muscle Diet,* you can go after any one of them, or you can collect the whole set, since they're by no means mutually exclusive. Each requires its own strategy. But, as you'll see, the strategies are designed to work together.

The Body You Want, for as Long as You Want It

In most body-transformation programs, maintenance is an afterthought. In *The Lean Muscle Diet,* it's the starting point. You begin at the end, with your final goal: maintaining a lean, athletic, muscular physique for life. You build your diet around your target body weight. That way, when you get there, you're already eating the right foods, in the right amounts, to maintain that weight. Same with the workouts: You'll start and finish with a schedule you can follow for life.

The most important phrase in the book is "as if." Success in many of life's most important endeavors begins with a commitment to act like the person you hope to become. This makes perfect sense if the subject is work or family. Your career path typically begins by getting the education your future employers expect you to have. At school you learn to think, speak, and eventually act like someone in your field. It works the same way in relationships. If you don't act like a guy in a relationship—being where you're supposed to be when you're supposed to be there, and rolling with the inevitable ups and downs of a shared life that's only partially within your control—you won't last long with that person.

And yet, when it comes to diet and exercise, the advice is rarely so practical and sustainable. Weight loss diets typically start with a massive reduction in daily calories, or by telling you to stop eating foods that you can't realistically avoid for long. Some, like the hideous "cleanse" diets, do both: They force you to stop eating altogether for a week or two. Unless you consider masochism an important life skill, these diets offer nothing useful.

Exercise, unlike eating, is a choice. It's a great choice; you'd be hard-pressed to find a credible expert who disagrees. But with so many ways to avoid it, it's tough to put together a routine that works for your body and fits into your life without interfering with something else. That's why it's so important to begin with that schedule, rather than one that's too ambitious to maintain or too lax to give you the results you want now and the structure to maintain them down the road.

For all those reasons, you'll act as if you're the guy you want to be from the first day of the Lean Muscle Plan.

"And You Are . . . ?"

Seems like a good time for introductions. The information about food and diet comes from my coauthor, Alan Aragon. I first met Alan in 2008 at a fitness event in Little Rock, Arkansas, where we were both doing presentations. I had no idea what to expect from him, since nutritionists at fitness conferences tend to fall into two camps.

- ▶ Fully invested in the conventional wisdom, and dry as cracked asphalt in August
- ▶ Fully invested in an unproven or disproven theory, and Mayan-apocalypse bonkers

Alan was his own category. He was an equal-opportunity debunker. He had no use for either the conventional wisdom or the stuff out on the edges.

He was the first person I heard use "broscience" to describe the urban legends passed down from lifelong gym rats to scrawny newbs. But debunking, fun as it is, doesn't really help anyone get bigger, stronger, or leaner. For that you need practical, actionable advice, and Alan delivered. I took pages of notes from that first presentation, and from every presentation I've seen him deliver since. I knew that the next time I wrote a book with a substantial diet emphasis, he was my first choice as coauthor.

You'll see Alan's plan in Part Two. It tells you exactly how to calculate your daily calorie needs, how to divide those calories into the number of meals you prefer to eat each day, and how to choose the best foods for your goals. And if anybody understands your goals, it's Alan. He started his career as a personal trainer before getting his nutrition degrees and certifications. So while he's as dedicated as anyone I know to digging through the current research, he never loses sight of what his clients and readers want from his knowledge and expertise: *results*. He works hard to find the information that will measurably improve your weight, body-fat percentage, or performance. Then he tests it and tweaks it and tests it again with individual clients until he finds systems and guidelines that work for most of the people who try them.

Me, I don't work one-on-one with clients the way Alan does. But I'm in touch with readers of my books and articles every day, and have been since my first book, *The Testosterone Advantage Plan,* came out in 2002. That book was inspired by my realization that many guys who wanted to lose weight were going about it wrong. Or, if not *wrong,* they were taking the scenic route when research pointed toward a faster, more direct path. Each subsequent book—*Home Workout Bible*; *Book of Muscle*; and the five books in the *New Rules of Lifting* series—was an attempt to answer questions asked by readers of the one I'd just published.

The Lean Muscle Diet takes me back to the beginning. It's inspired by what I see and hear from people who haven't yet learned the basic principles of strength training. The guys I see in gyms or interact with online remind me of myself in my teens and early adulthood. If you're one of them, you want what I wanted. But like me back then, you don't yet know what you don't know. You're sweating and grunting your way toward a dead end.

From the outside, it seems easy enough to act as if you're already an experienced lifter. You can join the same gym, wear the same clothes, follow the same schedule. But the illusion ends the minute you try to lift like one. It's like showing up at a law firm and sitting at a lawyer's desk. You might look like a lawyer, but as soon as you're expected to act like one, to offer the kind of advice that would keep someone out of trouble, or secure the least painful penalty for someone who already effed up, the world can see you're just pretending. You can't truly act as if you're a lawyer or a lifter until you know how to think like one.

For a lifter, you need to start with an understanding of how your body works, and how to make it work better. Only then can you begin to make it look better. Appearance is a result of performance. In Part Three, you'll learn how to get both results.

How to Use *The Lean Muscle Diet*

One thing I've learned in my long career as a fitness author: Few people start reading on page 1 and keep reading to the end. Most jump around. That's why Alan and I went into this with the idea that different readers will start with whatever part of the book is most important to them.

If you want to understand why our diet and workout plans are designed the way they are, and how they set you up for long-term success, please read Part One. That is, start at the beginning. We won't be offended if you're in a hurry to get to the programs, but we hope you circle back to the opening chapters when you get a chance.

If you're mostly concerned with your weight or body-fat percentage, the diet plan is in Part Two. The instructions are straightforward; all you need is a calculator. But if you get there and find yourself wondering why you have to do any math at all because you read somewhere that calories don't matter, you'll understand why it's a good idea to start at the beginning.

If you're mostly interested in the workout plan, you can go straight to Part Three. You can probably do okay with the workouts if you have some lifting experience. But it's better if you start out with an understanding of the choices that went into the program. For example, if you're wondering why the workouts train your entire body each time (and thus why there's no "arm day"), it would help to read the chapters that explain it. But the program should work for just about anybody who gives it a shot, since it's based on some of the oldest and most widely accepted concepts about increasing strength and size.

There are two other ways you might use this book: If you're just looking for healthy meal options or for new exercises to mix and match in your current workouts, you'll find plenty here—food choices in Part Two, exercises in Part Three.

But, whether you're trying to lose weight, gain weight, or keep your weight the same (only with less fat and more muscle), you'll have the most success by using *The Lean Muscle Diet*'s eating plan and workouts in tandem. Alan's diet provides exactly what you need to build muscle and fuel your workouts, while the training program gives your body the stimulus it needs to get leaner and stronger.

Best of all, at that point in the near or distant future when you look, move, and feel like a lifter, and someone asks you why so few people have been able to achieve results like yours, you can tell them the truth. "Because it's hard," you'll say. Then you'll add the all-important qualifier: "But not impossible."

And then, if they're still interested, you can explain to them what you're about to learn.

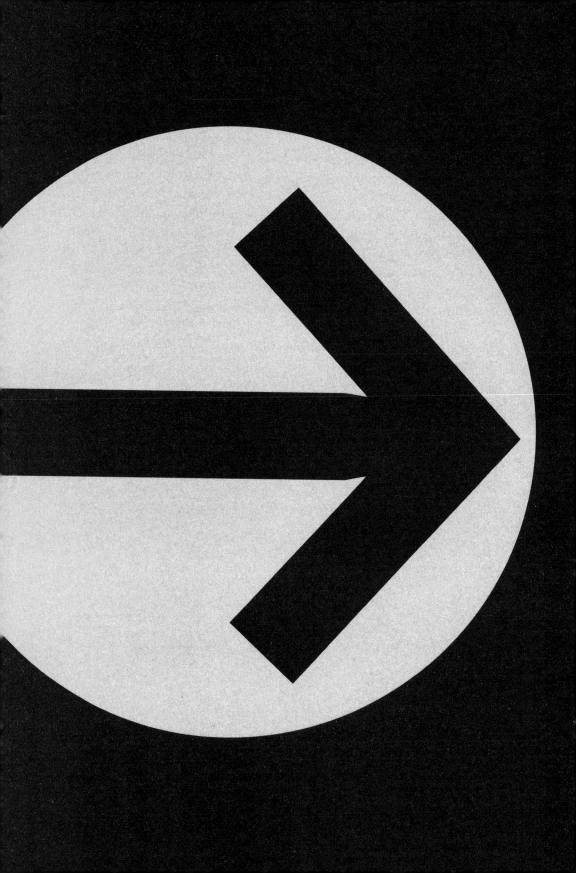

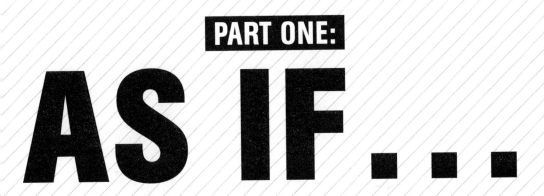

PART ONE:
AS IF....

CHAPTER 1

WHAT IF EVERYTHING YOU'VE BEEN TOLD IS TRUE?

LET'S SAY IT'S JANUARY 1. Strange as it seems, you wake up without a hangover—maybe because you don't drink, maybe because you're a doctor who just worked a holiday shift in the ER. (Hey, we don't judge.) Or maybe it's because you decided *this* is the year you're going to follow through on that resolution. The one to lose weight and get in shape. The one you've made 6 of the past 7 years, a streak that was broken up only by that time you were too depressed about your weight to think long term.

Anyway, it's going to happen this year. Totally. All you need is a plan.

Onetwothree go!

You Google "weight loss + doesn't suck." You check out the best-selling diet books on Amazon or at your local Barnes & Noble. You scroll through your Facebook feed. You ask your friends who don't seem to struggle with their weight. And what you get is . . . bewildering.

Over here you have one group that says calories don't matter. That's a relief, because with all the stuff you have to keep track of in your life, the last thing you want to do is obsess over every bite of food you take in.

When you dig in a little deeper, you see that the people telling you not to count calories are all-in on low-carb dieting. No bread, no cereals, no potatoes, no fruit. You're jolted back to your middle-school health class. On the one day you managed to stay awake, the teacher listed all those things as part of a healthy diet.

But here's another way to avoid counting. The paleo diet is all about eating like our ancient ancestors, before that evil thing called agriculture was invented. This diet makes a bit more sense to you. You can eat all the meat you want, along with fruits, vegetables, and nuts. But some of the rules still strike you as arbitrary. No beans? No grains of any kind? No dairy? You understand why cavemen wouldn't have eaten those things, and with 30 seconds of research you learn that the ability to digest milk into adulthood didn't exist until a few thousand years ago. But since it exists *now,* along with enzymes to help you digest grains, you're not sure why those foods are off-limits.

Yet another branch of the low-carb tribe seems obsessed with wheat in general, and gluten in particular. You aren't sure what gluten is, but you don't like the sound of it. It reminds you of the time you touched a blob of superglue and ended up with your thumb and forefinger stuck together. You spent the day giving complete strangers the OK sign. So that was unpleasant. As for gluten, you learn that it's mostly in bread, along with lots of snack foods you should avoid anyway. But it's also in . . . beer? Seriously? Well, so much for the thought of going gluten-free.

But what's this over here? This group isn't down on gluten at all. And they say you can eat all the food you want . . . as long as it's super-low in fat, and comes entirely from foods that never had a pulse. You can tolerate some vegetables, as long as they're in a salad and doused in dressing. But no meat, no dairy, no eggs? What's the point of eating a sandwich if you can't figure out what to put on the bread?

The more you search, the more confused you get. The only thing these groups have in common is passion. And in general you're pro-passion (except when it's from that ex-girlfriend who posted all those videos after you broke up with her). But whose passion will help *you* achieve *your* goals?

They all sound like they know what they're talking about. They all have rosters of authors and scientists and bloggers who agree with them. They cite published research that, to them, is persuasive evidence that they're right and everyone else is living in a fantasy world. You're left with one overwhelming impression: If any of them is right, then all the rest are wrong. How in the world does a regular guy with a job and a life figure out which is which?

It Gets Worse

All you've gotten out of your research so far is an empty stomach. But you still have no idea what you should or shouldn't eat. So you decide to put the whole diet thing on hold while you eat some leftover pizza and find a workout plan for the new year. This should be easier, right? Your goal is to take off fat and put on muscle. Surely everyone agrees on the best way to do that.

As the man said, get used to disappointment.

Some sources swear by cardio exercise for weight loss, but you know that's not for you. Your previous attempts at weight loss via exercise have proved beyond a reasonable doubt that you're not a runner, swimmer, cyclist, rower, or triathlete.

Good thing there's another camp to tell you that cardio exercise is unnecessary. Some even go so far as to say it's *bad* for you. It eats up your muscle tissue like tapeworms and leaves you with nothing but deep fatigue and battered knees. At the farthest fringes a few even claim that cardio makes you sick and fat.

That doesn't make any sense. The runners you know are lean and healthy. You just know you're not one of them. But at the same time, the anti-cardio camp appeals to you for the simple reason that the muscular physique you want can only be achieved with strength training.

Alas, there seems to be no agreement about the best way to build it. You find a group that says you just need to lift three times a week for 20 minutes at a time. It sounds too good to be true, and with one glance at the fine print, you see it is. You do just one set of each exercise, but you can't stop the set until you reach a point where your muscles are completely, painfully exhausted. It sounds more like self-torture than self-improvement.

So you keep looking. You find bodybuilders who recommend training five or six times a week, with specialized workouts for every muscle group, large or small. You find experts who want you to do everything with a barbell, or kettlebells, or nylon straps hanging from a chinup bar, or elastic bands, or your own body weight, or something else. And then there's CrossFit, which turned exercise into a sport, with a combination of gymnastics movements and Olympic lifts. CrossFitters give you the impression that any workout without vomit is a wasted opportunity; you should've just stayed home and manscaped your eyebrows.

Similar to the diet evangelists, each fitness camp believes it's right. And not just right: They're absolutely, unequivocally right, which means every-one who disagrees with their methods, in whole or in part, is absolutely, unequivocally wrong. They overwhelm you with studies and testimonials to support their positions.

All this is aside from the factions you dismissed at first glance: the ones who say exercise is a waste of time because it just makes you hungry; the calorie-restriction cultists who think they'll live longer by starving them-selves; and the well-meaning enthusiasts who are so into something—yoga, Spinning, Prancercise—that they imagine it offers all kinds of benefits you find unlikely.

Now, like millions before you, you wonder if anyone can give you what you want: diet and workout plans that make sense, that work together, that aren't based on magic or faith, and that a regular guy with a busy life can do. Oh, and it would be nice if they actually work.

As luck would have it . . .

The Truth about Truth

Alan and I have a radical proposition for you: *Everybody is right.* All the dif-ferent diet and exercise camps, no matter how contradictory they seem and how loud they scream about how wrong everyone else is, are saying basically the same two things.

1. If you want to change your weight, in either direction, you must find a way to create an imbalance between the calories you take in and the calories you expend.

When we talk about how to gain weight, everyone agrees on this principle. Of course you have to *eat* bigger if you want to *be* bigger. But for some reason it's controversial when we talk about weight loss. Here's what's funny: The peo-ple who argue against this basic rule of weight control—and a lot of them these days say calories don't matter—are among the very best at finding ways for people to eat less total food. That's the biggest benefit of any weight loss diet: It gives you a systematic way to both account for and reduce the number of calories you eat on a daily basis.

How they do it is no mystery.

- ▶ Low-carb diets, like Atkins or paleo, tell you to avoid the foods that many of us overeat when given the chance. Personally, I find it very hard to stop at a couple slices of pizza when that third one is just sitting right there, the scent of garlic, baked bread, and melted cheese shamelessly taunting me. Same with pancakes or doughnuts or even a really good sandwich. It's easier just to avoid them altogether.

- ▶ Low-fat diets, including vegetarian or vegan, get you to avoid the foods with the highest caloric density—the ones that give you the most calories in each serving.

- ▶ Most weight loss diets rule out any type of "food" that requires a one-syllable modifier like "fast," "snack," or "junk." They get you to eat whole or minimally processed foods, most of which require some preparation. Everyone agrees that this is the healthiest way to eat, and in *The Lean Muscle Diet* it's probably the most important part of Alan's system.

- ▶ To replace those highly processed foods, low-carb and paleo-inspired diets get you to eat more protein. Throughout *The Lean Muscle Diet* we'll tell you in exhaustive detail exactly why protein is the key to your two most important outcomes: building muscle and losing fat.

- ▶ Vegetarian and vegan diets get you to eat shit-tons of vegetables, which are packed with fiber, which means you shit tons. Paleo and other low-carb diets also tend to include a lot of vegetables, for basically the same reason.

- ▶ One other benefit to eating lots of vegetables: Like protein, they help you feel full faster during a meal, and retain that feeling longer between meals. Both of those outcomes—satiety and satiation—help with the big goal of eating less, and thus creating an imbalance between the calories coming in and those going out.

- ▶ Diets based on fasting seem to help enthusiasts reduce calories by limiting the hours in which you can eat. A popular system requires you to fast 16 hours a day (including 8 hours of sleep), and then eat whatever you want in the remaining time. Fasting isn't for me; I'm a lifelong breakfast eater who rarely goes more than 4 or 5 waking hours without food. But on the anecdotal level, you'll find lots of support for the idea that eating less frequently correlates with eating less food.

2. If you want to build more muscle than you have now, you need to get stronger.

To your body, muscle is both a necessity and a luxury. It's necessary to get you where you need to go to obtain food and water. But throughout human history, there were enormous differences in the food-retrieving challenges faced by populations in different parts of the world.

So our ancient ancestors developed different sets of traits to thrive in their individual environments. Some were small-framed because they needed to travel long distances through deserts or over mountains. For them even a few extra pounds of muscle would have been a burden—more weight to haul through deserts or over mountains, and a hungry source of calories that were difficult to obtain. Some were thick-framed because they needed strength to hunt and insulation to survive long winters. The extra fat they carried also provided a source of fuel when they failed to bring home a caribou or seal or whatever they were hunting that day. They needed more muscle to support the extra bulk, but only to a point. Meanwhile, people in temperate climates developed frames that were somewhere in between. The available evidence suggests they would have been leaner than most of us today, but they certainly wouldn't have looked like a modern bodybuilder. Nobody needed that much muscle to get through the day, and you have to suppose that few people could afford to feed an extravagantly muscled body.

As it happens, most of us have genes from multiple environments. Our ancestors moved around; their genes mixed and matched and randomly mutated, just because they could. We developed all kinds of traits that have nothing to do with survival.

Today most of us spend the majority of our time sitting. You don't need a lot of muscle to transport you from your car to your office and back to your car again, with a handful of unhurried strolls to the restroom in between. But, thanks to first-world affluence, most of you reading this can afford to feed all the muscle mass you can grow. Moreover, muscle that's excessive relative to our foraging needs isn't necessarily a luxury. It provides us with a long list of health benefits, along with the obvious boost to our self-confidence and the potential mating opportunities that go along with it. (See "Special Topic: What Women Want," on page 10.)

Strength training makes your muscles bigger through three basic processes:

1. Mechanical tension. You perform exercises that are challenging to your muscles, connective tissues, and bones. The work has to be hard, but not so hard it tears them apart. You do this repeatedly and systematically. Your body responds to the challenge by increasing the size and strength of the tissues.

2. Metabolic stress. You can build muscle with heavy weights, light weights, and everything in between. But when you're using lighter weights, it's important to make sure you take your muscles to a deep level of exhaustion. That triggers a hormonal cascade that's linked to muscle growth.

3. Muscle damage. A good workout will create small disruptions in the muscle fibers. You don't need to feel muscle damage for it to take place, much less work out in a way that guarantees soreness, or leaves you so stiff you make the zombies in *Night of the Living Dead* look like a clip from *Dancing with the Stars*. It's simply a side effect of a solid training program, one that results in bigger, stronger muscles.

Looking at these three ways to stimulate muscle growth, you may wonder how they support my original point: that you have to make muscles stronger to make them bigger. It's because the first one—mechanical tension—is by far the most important driver of muscle growth. The key to mechanical tension is *progressive overload*. You make your body do more work over time in a systematic way. Strength increases, and muscle mass follows.

That said, the link between strength and size isn't entirely straightforward. If this is your first program, your strength will probably increase much faster than your mass. And elite athletes in weight-class sports have made an art and science out of increasing strength without getting bigger.

But it remains the most reliable way we know of to increase the size of your muscles, just as controlling the number of calories you eat is the only guaranteed way to change your weight in either direction.

That's what we'll tackle in Chapter 2.

WHAT WOMEN WANT

IF YOU BUILD IT, THEY WILL . . . WELL, YOU KNOW

Many years ago I had a conversation with the editor of *Muscle & Fitness* magazine. He showed me a black-and-white picture of the biggest bodybuilder I had ever seen. The editor told me the physique represented his personal aesthetic, and what he thought his readers aspired to. To me the guy looked like a rockslide with nipples.

Muscle & Fitness in the mid-1990s was a deeply weird magazine in lots of ways. To pick just one, there was what I called the magazine's Big Lie: The more muscle you have, the more women will be attracted to you. I figured my future colleagues at *Men's Health* magazine had the right idea with their cover models. They understood that genetically average guys like me would be inspired by a physique that's just a bit bigger and leaner than we could ever hope to attain.

But here's a question none of us could answer back then: What type of physique did *women* find most attractive? The scientific evidence has coalesced around a few basic ideas. Facial symmetry, for example, suggests reproductive health. Which is nice to know, but unless you're born into the symmetrical elite, it would take some really expensive surgery to make your eyes or ears match up. (And even then you'd probably end up looking like a space alien.)

Some studies postulated that women tend to go for the most masculine-looking guys when they're ovulating (and thus more likely to get pregnant); at other times they prefer guys who offer more nurturing qualities. From that you'd suppose women would prefer more muscular, athletic-looking guys for short-term affairs, including hookups and one-nighters, but not for more serious relationships.

But how do you test that?

In a study published in 2007, UCLA researchers asked young women for information about their real-life sexual encounters. The result: "Women were more willing to have short-term relations with muscular men without the requirement that they demonstrate characteristics particularly desired in long-term mates."

I learned about this body of research when I was asked to work on an article for *Men's Health* on the golden ratio, a proportion of length to width that comes out to 1.6. Leonardo applied the ratio to many of his paintings and designs (as he explained in his best-selling memoir, *The Da Vinci Code*). Turns out, women are most attracted to a V-shaped torso, which includes shoulders that are 60 percent wider than the waist. That was the conclusion of research by University of Westminster psychologist Viren Swami, PhD, whom I interviewed for the article. Since it's awkward to measure the circumference of your shoulders, you can use your chest girth instead. In that case, the ideal ratio would be 1.4—a chest that's 40 percent larger than your waist.

But there's some important fine print. "An obese man with the ideal ratio would probably be perceived as unattractive," Swami told me in an e-mail. It's also important to keep in mind the phrase "all else being equal." "Romantic relationships and interpersonal attraction are extremely complicated," he said. It'll never be as simple as writing up a list and finding exactly what you want in the relationships aisle of Trader Joe's.

The best reason to get in shape and stay in shape is because of what it does for you. When you look better you feel better, and when you feel better you look better. If that means more opportunities to make a good first impression, consider it a welcome side effect.

CHAPTER 2:

WHAT MAKES A DIET WORK

BEFORE YOU CAN FULLY APPRECIATE why a diet works, it helps to understand why the last one *didn't*. Or, I should say, why the last one worked for a while but then stopped. Why it worked at first is no mystery: Just about everything does, as you saw in Chapter 1. Despite different methods and rationales, *they all do the same basic thing*: They get you to eat less. The math always works.

The problem begins with *how* they get you to eat less. Most of them demonize some type of food. It could be a single food, like wheat or dairy, or it could be an entire macronutrient, like fat or carbohydrates. Since there are only three macronutrients—protein is the third—eliminating one of them means a huge percentage of the food chain is off-limits to you for as long as you stick with the diet. Which probably won't be long, if the diet is too restrictive.

But what does that even mean? We all understand that a healthy diet has to restrict *something*. What it should restrict, and how much, and how often, are the questions that divide us. So let's see if we can agree on some diet guidelines that give us the best shot at building a lean, athletic, healthy body, preferably one that we can maintain without a lifetime of suffering.

Quantity Matters

Calories are units of energy. And *energy balance,* over time, determines whether you gain or lose mass. The *type* of mass you gain or lose is determined by lots of factors, which we'll explain as we go along. But when you're trying to change the *amount* of mass—the solid tissue that includes your muscle, organs, fat, and bones—the outcome depends on your ability to manage energy coming in versus energy going out.

In the short term, all kinds of issues can mask your body's actual energy balance. The most frustrating one, when you're trying to lose weight, is water. Water is between 45 and 65 percent of your weight—less if you have a lot of fat (fat cells have very little), more if you're lean. Your muscles are about 75 percent water, as is your brain and most of your organs. The total amount can fluctuate by a couple pounds from day to day, but it's not especially important when we're talking about long-term energy balance.

Which we are.

The problem with energy balance is that it's complicated. But it's hard to spur humans to take action unless you present things as stark choices. So well-meaning public-health officials pretend that the solution to obesity is simply "eat less, move more." In an earlier generation, fitness guru Jack LaLanne used to describe food as "ten seconds on the lips, a lifetime on the hips." They score some pithiness points, but not many for accuracy. Let's walk through the actual steps of human metabolism and see what their bumper-sticker slogans leave out.

> **1. Calories in:** You eat something. So far, so good.
>
> **2. Calories out:** On average, about 10 percent of all the food you eat will be burned up during digestion, which we call the *thermic effect of food,* or TEF. But the total varies with the content of the meal. The TEF for protein is about 25 percent. That means a quarter of the protein you eat disappears before it reaches your muscles. For fat it's just 2 to 3 percent, and for carbs it's 6 to 8 percent.
>
> Already we've found a potential exception to the "eat less" half of the slogan. If you eat less protein, you actually make it *harder* to lose weight. And if you replace some fat and carbohydrates with protein, you should make it easier to lose weight, even if you eat the same amount of food overall.
>
> **3. More calories out:** You also lose some energy with the things we don't discuss in polite company: urine, gas, feces.

It's not a huge amount, and Alan on his worst day wouldn't give you a diet that increased your methane output. But it's important to note that "a lifetime on the hips" doesn't apply to the small percentage of foods that go in one end and out the other, bypassing the hips entirely.

What's left after steps 2 and 3 is *metabolizable energy* (a phrase that'll get you absolutely nowhere with the ladies). Those calories are dealt with in the next two steps.

4. *More* calories out: Now your body begins the work of keeping you alive. Breathing. Pumping blood. Breaking down and building up your body at the cellular level. Thinking. (Your brain, which is about 2 percent of your body mass, uses 20 percent of your total energy.) This is called your *basal* or *resting metabolism,* and it can account for as much as 70 percent of the energy you expend each day.

Your body's lean tissue—everything that isn't fat—is the driver of your basal metabolism. The more you have, all else being equal, the more calories you need just to keep it all going.

5. *Even more* calories out: Now we get to voluntary physical activity—moving around, exercising, maybe occasionally having sex. For most of us, this will be about 20 to 30 percent of our daily energy expenditure.

To review: Between step 1 ("calories in") and step 5 (movement you do on purpose), you have three incredibly important steps that account for 70 to 80 percent of the total calories you burn each day. So while it's simple to tell people to "eat less, move more," the truth is that the moment you do either one, all the steps in between change. When you eat less, your body burns less in steps 2, 3, 4, and 5. And when you move more on a regular basis, you'll probably end up eating more, which changes step 1. And that, yet again, changes what happens in steps 2 through 5, although not necessarily for the worse.

But just because your body has all these *involuntary* ways to manipulate your metabolism doesn't mean you can't impose *voluntary* upgrades. Eating more protein will have the biggest impact in the short term, and we'll say a lot about that later in this chapter. Strength training is the biggest one in the long term, since it gives you a mechanism to not only burn calories while you do it, but also to burn more chronically as you add to your body's lean mass. You'll hear plenty about that as well.

So what's the right quantity of food? Alan's take, as you already know, is to eat enough to maintain the body you want to have. If that body has less mass than You 1.0, you need to eat less. If You 2.0 is bigger than the beta version, you need to eat more. You'll find the exact numbers in Chapter 5. For now, let's move on to the next-most-important factor in a successful diet.

Quality Matters

In a simpler, more innocent time, we would have said this one is a no-brainer. *Of course* the quality of your diet is important. That's why health professionals still talk about food groups and "balanced" diets. But around the time we stopped using "no-brainer," we realized we can't talk about quality without defining it. Which is trickier than it sounds.

In a review that came out in 2009, Australian researchers identified 25 different systems for ranking diet quality used in published studies. Most of them were based on nutrients (vitamins, minerals, fiber, etc.), foods or food groups (grains, meat, vegetables, and so on), or some combination of the two. The review concluded, to no one's surprise, that the people with the best diets live the longest and are least likely to die of cardiovascular disease. It didn't seem to matter which index of quality was used.

Alas, studies like these tell us less than we think. The results are only as good as the data they're based on. The data comes from people filling out surveys based on their memories of what they ate and how much. Not only is human memory flawed, it's *human*. That means it's biased in favor of what people think they're supposed to eat. We end up with conventional wisdom that coalesces around flawed ideas, like the notion that animal fats are "bad," and therefore vegetable fats must be better. A generation of Americans followed that advice by using margarine instead of butter ... until we learned that the fats in margarine are the ones most likely to cause heart disease. Oops!

The "Whole" Truth

Fortunately, there aren't many food fights that end up with a body count. The arguments get heated, with occasional flecks of spittle released, but you won't die if you bet on the wrong definition of a healthy diet. Since most diets do the same things, as we've been saying, the benefits of using them successfully should be similar as well.

To Alan, a quality diet looks like this.

- ▶ 80 percent whole and minimally processed foods you like

- ▶ 10 percent whole and minimally processed foods you don't necessarily like, but don't hate

- ▶ 10 percent whatever you want—"pure junky goodness," as Alan likes to say

Careful readers will note the key phrase: "whole and minimally processed." Not all processing is bad. Cooking, for example, is a type of processing. It usually makes the nutrients in the food more bioavailable than they are in raw form. Cooking also lowers the risk that bacterial nasties can attack you from the inside. On top of all that, cooking almost always makes the food taste better (carrots being an obvious exception).

The problems with processing begin when the food is *substantially* altered to the point where it's impossible to look at it and tell what it once was. Take wheat, for example. Before it can become white bread or a delicious piecrust, two parts of the wheat kernel must be removed. First to go is the outer layer, called the bran. This is the part with most of the fiber, along with protein, fat, iron, and some vitamins. Next to go is the germ, which is the reproductive center of the kernel. Although it's a small part of the grain, it's rich in protein and fat. That leaves the endosperm. It's almost all carbohydrate. But that's good from a commercial viewpoint. Without the fats in the germ, which would eventually turn rancid, the resulting flour will last for years. And without the bran, the flour is white, which in a bygone time was considered preferable to brown flour, the default nutrition of the poor and starving. Sometimes the white flour is bleached to make it even whiter. If a food label says the flour was "enriched," that means vitamins and minerals were added back in. What's left is a product that doesn't look like, taste like, or offer the nutritional profile of the original food.

On the other hand, you have protein powders. Most are made from milk proteins, but they don't look or taste like milk, and the proteins are typically separated. So while dairy protein is 80 percent casein and just 20 percent whey, the protein supplements you buy are far more likely to be all or mostly whey. Moreover, the least essential part of the milk—a sugar called lactose, which is problematic for many—is usually removed. What you have left is a highly processed nutritional supplement with a long list of proven or proposed health benefits. The main one is its role in building and supporting muscle—the reason most of us use it, and why Alan recommends it in Part Two. Recent research shows that whey may also help with weight loss, blood-sugar management, and disease prevention.

So when Alan uses "whole and minimally processed" as a category, what he really means is this: "foods that aren't classic junk food." So you have the obvious choices.

▶ Flesh from land and sea animals

▶ Milk

▶ Eggs

▶ Nuts and seeds

▶ Fruits

▶ Vegetables

▶ Potatoes and other tubers

▶ Legumes (a category that includes peas, beans, lentils, and peanuts)

Then you have judgment-call choices, which have undergone some processing but still provide useful nutrients.

▶ Dairy products like cheese and yogurt

▶ Whole grain products like bread and cereal

▶ Refined-grain products like white rice, which are staples in the diets of some of the healthiest people in the world

At the end of the list are supplemental foods like protein powders and some of the others Alan recommends in Chapter 6. All of these fit in the 90 percent of your diet that is "whole and minimally processed."

Part of that 90 percent—10 percent of your total calories—will come from "whole and minimally processed foods you don't necessarily like, but don't hate." Alan includes this for the simple reason that few guys will hit their daily targets for fruits and vegetables without being told they have to. We have substantial evidence that those foods, eaten regularly and with as little processing as possible, protect us against heart disease and cancer, the two leading causes of death in the United States. We also know that vitamin and mineral pills are a poor substitute for the real thing. (We'll have much more on this later in the chapter.) Whole foods provide benefits you can't get with isolated nutrients.

In other words, this is where you eat your spinach.

In Defense of the Indefensible

Ten percent of your calories will come from Alan's "pure junky goodness" category. It doesn't really require explanation, but I'd be remiss if I didn't share Alan's take in all its glory:

"Dietary perfection is a myth. It doesn't exist. There is no Unicorn Diet for humans. (Although it's entirely possible that someone will read that sentence and come up with one.) Ten percent of the diet coming from anything you want might sound rebellious until you switch things around and see that 90 percent of the diet is a diligent effort to cover all the bases, which in all candidness is a soup of uncertainty on its own."

For social proof, Alan dug up these dietary tidbits from the world's longest-living humans (we boldfaced our favorite details).

> Sarah DeRemer Clark-Knauss was 119 when she died in 1999.
> She was married for 64 years, and still managed to outlive
> her husband by 34 years: "She was born in Hollywood,
> Pennsylvania, a small coal-mining town which no longer exists.
> **She loved chocolate.** She died in Allentown, Pennsylvania, in
> the nursing home, which she had lived in for 9 years. She never
> had a full-time job, but was a homemaker and insurance-office
> manager."

> Jeanne Louise Calment was 122 when she died in 1997, and
> claimed to have met Vincent van Gogh in France in 1888:
> "Calment ascribed her longevity and relatively youthful

appearance for her age to a diet rich in olive oil, and rubbed onto her skin, as well as a diet of port wine, and ate **nearly 1 kilogram (2.2 pounds) of chocolate every week.** Calment reportedly remained mentally intact until her very end."

Salustiano Sanchez-Blazquez was 112 when he died in 2013: "Sanchez-Blazquez had said his longevity was attributed to eating **one banana per day and his daily dose of six Anacin tablets.** His daughter had another theory. 'I think it's just because he's an independent, stubborn man,' she said."

George Johnson was also 112 when he died in 2006: "'He had terrible bad habits. **He had a diet largely of sausages and waffles,**' Dr. L. Stephen Coles, founder of the Gerontology Research Group at the University of California, Los Angeles, said Friday."

Here's the only fine print in Alan's plan: The 10 percent guideline doesn't necessarily mean 10 percent of your food *every day*. Let's say the calculations in Chapter 5 suggest you eat 2,500 daily calories to reach your target weight. That's 17,500 calories a week. Ten percent of those—1,750 calories—are up for grabs. Many of Alan's clients like to use them up each day, giving them 250 calories for a candy bar or small dessert. But some prefer the big bang of a cheat meal, saving all 1,750 for a single blowout. Or you can do anything in between.

You don't need a nutrition expert to tell you what qualifies for this category. If Twinkies still exist when you read this, they go here, along with:

▶ Sugar-sweetened beverages (sodas, sports drinks, commercial iced teas)

▶ Ice cream and frozen desserts

▶ Baked goods (cookies, cakes, pies)

▶ Anything you'd serve with syrup or reasonably describe as "dessert for breakfast"

▶ Candy (although, based on the longevity stories, you have to wonder if chocolate is tragically misclassified)

▶ French fries and anything else breaded and deep-fried

Protein Matters

You know protein is the stuff muscles are made of. Or, more accurately, after you take away the 75 percent that's water, most of what's left is protein. (About 1 percent is carbohydrate, in the form of glycogen, and there's a bit of fat and salt in there as well.) And it's not just your muscles: Protein makes up about 20 percent of your body's mass. Not only is it the key structural component of your cells, it also forms your hormones and enzymes and allows cells throughout your body to communicate with each other. It comprises your hair, your blood, and your fingernails and toenails. These cells break down and rebuild themselves all day, every day.

Your body, interestingly, can recycle that broken-down protein, a survival mechanism that would have helped our ancestors through an unlucky stretch of hunting and gathering. You'll die with no protein at all, but you can live for a long time with minimal amounts.

That recycling mechanism is why protein recommendations from the government and mainstream nutrition organizations tend to be much lower than what most of us eat without even trying. It's also why a nutritionist will be quick to tell you that no one needs as much protein as Alan recommends in *The Lean Muscle Diet*. Alan will be just as quick to ask how the nutritionist defines "needs." If you're talking about the needs of a person who's mostly sedentary and isn't trying to lose weight or build muscle, minimal amounts work just fine.

But when you add strength training to the mix, forget about minimalism. Now you're deliberately increasing the rate of muscle-protein breakdown, with the goal of creating new muscle tissue at an even higher rate. Logically, that requires more protein from your diet.

Now add another element: a lower-calorie diet. The diet puts stress on your muscle tissue in two ways. First, it gives your body less overall energy to support the process of muscle repair and growth. Second, that protein in your muscles can become a source of energy when you're eating below maintenance levels. The leaner you are, the smaller your margin for error before your body turns to muscle tissue for fuel.

Researchers who study athletes and bodybuilders have found that the harder you train, the more disciplined your diet, and the leaner you are, the more protein you need to avoid losing muscle along with fat. Here's what the continuum looks like, in chart form. On the left side, Alan starts with the US government's Recommended Dietary Allowance (RDA); on the right side, he shows the higher levels recommended by studies.

PROTEIN INTAKE CONTINUUM	
LOWER PROTEIN NEEDS: 0.8–1.2 GRAMS PER KILOGRAM* OF BODY WEIGHT PER DAY	HIGHER PROTEIN NEEDS: 1.6–2.7 GRAMS PER KILOGRAM OF BODY WEIGHT PER DAY
You're eating at or above maintenance	You're eating below maintenance
You're doing light exercise, without specific training goals	You're doing vigorous, progressive, goal-oriented training
You have moderate to high body fat	You have low body fat
You aren't trying to gain muscle	You're training to gain muscle, or at least preserve what you have while losing fat
Your doctor recommends a low-protein diet for medical reasons	You have no medical restrictions

*To keep the fractions from getting too ugly, we use kilograms instead of pounds. A kilogram is 2.2 pounds, so the lower end of recommended protein intake is 0.36 to 0.54 gram per pound per day, and the high end is 0.73 to 1.23 grams.

In Alan's plan, as you'll see in Chapter 5, he makes the math simple: You'll have 1 gram of protein per pound of target body weight per day. So if your target weight is 180 pounds, you'll shoot for 180 grams. That should give you plenty to build and repair muscle following your workouts, while also giving you a powerful tool to increase your metabolism and limit hunger.

The Best and Worst Proteins for Your Goals

Protein quality matters at least as much as quantity. Different foods have different combinations of 20 amino acids—the building blocks of protein—and some combinations are more potent than others. Nine of the 20 are considered "essential," meaning your body can't make them; they have to come from your diet. Of those nine, three are categorized as branched-chain amino acids (BCAAs). Leucine is the most powerful BCAA, and the single most important nutrient for building muscle.

Here's a quick look at which foods have the most BCAA in general, and leucine in particular, and which have the least.

PROTEIN SOURCE	BCAA	LEUCINE
Whey isolate	26%	14%
Milk (80% casein, 20% whey)	21%	10%
Egg	20%	8.5%
Animal flesh*	18%	8%
Soy isolate	18%	8%
Wheat	15%	7%

*This category includes the muscle tissue of cattle, pigs, birds, fish, and whatever else is in those mysterious chunks of organic matter we call fast food.

Whey protein is hands-down the best for building or preserving muscle. But whey is a supplement, and most of your daily calories should come from whole foods. That means you'll focus on the next three foods in the chart: dairy, eggs, and animal flesh (meat, poultry, fish). If you happen to be a vegetarian, you'll rely more on the two foods at the bottom of the chart, along with legumes like beans and lentils.

Carbohydrates Matter

Carbohydrates do one thing: provide energy. And if you look only at the broad outlines of human metabolism, you'd assume they do it pretty well. We noted earlier that your brain uses 20 percent of your daily energy—500 calories for a guy eating 2,500 calories a day. All of it comes from a sugar called glucose. No matter what type of carbohydrate you eat—bananas, fettuccine, Gummi Frogs—it all turns to glucose during digestion. From there it's the preferred fuel for both mind and muscles.

In fact, glucose is so important to your survival that your body doesn't trust carbohydrates to provide it. Through a process called *gluconeogenesis,* you can make glucose out of amino acids. (Leucine is one of the few aminos that can't be converted.) It seems to occur even when you have plenty of carbs in your diet.

So, in the most literal sense, carbohydrates *don't* matter for short-term survival. But they sure as hell matter in all practical ways. They're crucial to athletic performance, especially in endurance events but also, to a lesser extent, in sports like soccer and basketball, which require a mix of stamina and short bursts of speed and power.

The average American man's diet is about 48 percent carbs. Those who are classified as overweight and obese don't eat a higher percentage than those who are considered "normal" weight. (A full explanation of those categories awaits you in Chapter 4.) Think about that for a moment. While the heaviest people clearly eat the most food, it doesn't follow that they eat the highest proportion of carbs. Nor does it follow that cutting carbs is the best weight loss strategy for everyone, as Alan will explain in a moment.

Before we get there, let's clear up some definitional issues.

The Meaningless Classifications That Launched a Thousand Stupid Arguments

You've heard carbohydrates described as "simple" or "complex." I think they start teaching it to kids in third grade now. A simple carb has only one type of sugar. That sugar can be a *monosaccharide,* like glucose or fructose, or it can be a *disaccharide,* like sucrose, better known as table sugar, which combines glucose with fructose. Complex carbs are usually *polysaccharides*: long chains of sugar molecules.

Typically, if someone uses the word "complex" in front of "carbohydrate," it's to imply it's superior to a simple carb. Problem is, an apple is a simple carb, as are lots of healthy, nutritious foods. And white bread, long used as a worst-case example of food processing, is complex.

A better word for complex carbs is starch. Starches are found in most of the foods we eat: cereal grains (wheat, corn, rice, oats), tubers (potatoes, sweet potatoes, yams), and beans. Even bananas start out with some starch, which turns to glucose and fructose as they ripen. From that list of foods, you can't make any blanket statements about the nutritious qualities of starches. You find them in both the most and least processed foods, from pastries to baked potatoes.

Since we live in a carbophobic age, lots of people out there want to make these choices easy for you. Some diets, like Atkins, tell you to avoid almost all carbohydrates, no matter if they're simple or complex. Others, like paleo, make distinctions based on how long something has been a part of the human diet. Still others tell you that wheat is the problem. Shit will kill you, man!

Meanwhile, the longest-lived people in the world eat diets based on starches, as described in the book *Blue Zones,* by Dan Buettner. These include whole grains (on Ikaria, a Greek island); rice, beans, and corn (Nicoya, in Costa Rica); and barley and fava beans (Sardinia, an Italian island).

So if there's no meaningful distinction between simple and complex carbs, and if most people eat about the same percentage of carbohydrates whether they're fat or thin, there must be some better way to look at carbs, and to decide how to use them in our diets to get the results we want. As it turns out, there is.

"Because Insulin"

If your body were the US government, the hormone insulin would be the executive branch. You only think it runs the show because it gets the headlines. That's why insulin gets blamed for every ounce of fat that ends up on your love handles, and gets none of the credit for the important work it does to build your muscles and keep you from overeating.

We know that eating carbohydrates causes insulin to surge, and the more carbs you eat, the higher it goes. (Protein has a similar effect, but we don't often mention that.) When insulin levels are high, your body can't release stored energy from your fat cells, which means you're temporarily more dependent on using glucose for energy. That's not a problem in the short term. As noted earlier, your brain, neurons, and muscles run on glucose, and getting it directly from carbohydrates in your food is easier than making it from amino acids or taking it from the glycogen stored in your muscles and liver.

If you're healthy, your body will quickly return to a normal state, with the glucose successfully cleared from the bloodstream and your metabolism humming along on a mix of fuels that includes more fat than glucose. One way your body achieves that is with insulin. It acts as a powerful brake on your appetite while shuttling the food you just ate into the appropriate places—muscles, liver, fat cells.

Insulin gets a bad rap in fad diets because of that last thing: pushing excess nutrients—both fat and carbs—into fat cells. (And it gets too little credit for pushing protein into muscle cells, which is the reward for all your hard work in the gym.) But even that is no big deal. *Fat cells aren't prison cells.* Energy goes in and out all the time. It's only when you're eating more food than your body can use that you have to worry. That's not because of insulin—it's because you ate too damned much.

Clearly, though, some of us handle our carbs better than others. Put another way, some of us are more sensitive to the effects of insulin than others. That means we need less of it to sweep glucose from our bloodstream, and it works better as an appetite killer. A University of Colorado study, published in 2005, showed how insulin sensitivity can affect weight loss.

Women in the study were assigned a diet that was either low-carb (20 percent carbs, 60 percent fat) or low-fat (60 percent carbs, 20 percent fat). Both diets had 20 percent protein. The women classified as insulin-sensitive lost twice as much weight on the low-fat diet; those classified as insulin-resistant lost more on the low-carb diet.

There's only so much you can read into any single study (especially when you're a guy and the subjects are women), but in this case it matches what Alan and other weight loss specialists see pretty much every day. If you have a lot of weight to lose, and especially if you're a couple years behind on your workouts, you probably have some degree of insulin resistance. High-carb meals will create more problems for you than they will for someone who's leaner and has a higher fitness level.

Which is a perfect time to segue to the question of how much we should eat.

The Carbohydrate Continuum

A recent position stand by the International Society of Sports Nutrition suggests the following ranges for daily carb consumption. Keep in mind that these recommendations are for maximum performance, not for people who are most interested in getting leaner or reaching a specific weight.

ACTIVITY LEVEL	CARB NEEDS (SHOWN AS GRAMS PER KILOGRAM OF BODY WEIGHT PER DAY)
You're a regular guy working out several times a week	3–5 g/kg/day
You're a serious athlete training 2 to 3 hours a day, 5 to 6 days a week	5–8 g/kg/day
You're a pro athlete training 3 to 6 hours a day, 5 to 6 days a week	8–10 g/kg/day

Most *Lean Muscle Diet* readers will go with the recommendation on the top line. If you have a target body weight of 180 pounds (82 kilograms), you would shoot for about 250 daily grams of carbohydrates at the low end. Since carbs usually have 4 calories per gram (it varies by small amounts that aren't worth worrying about), you'd get about 1,000 calories per day. That's 40 percent of a 2,500-calorie diet. You're also getting about 30 percent of your calories from protein (180 grams × 4 calories per gram = 720 calories), which leaves 30 percent for fat. In other words, the classic 40:30:30 Zone diet.

But before we talk about fat, there's one more carbohydrate topic to cover.

Shit Happens, Thanks to Fiber

Fiber is the one type of carbohydrate that almost everyone agrees is beneficial. High-fiber foods, like fibrous vegetables, have relatively few calories, and the calories they have tend to serve a noble purpose. They either (a) keep food in your stomach longer—this slows down the surge of glucose in your blood, which in turn mutes the insulin response; or (b) speed up the transit of food through your system, which gives you bigger and more predictable bowel movements. The older you get, the more you appreciate those. (Trust me.)

Traditionally, fiber is classified as either soluble or insoluble in water. Soluble fiber is most often found in oats, barley, nuts, seeds, beans, lentils, peas, and some fruits and vegetables. It soaks up water in your stomach, forming a gel that stays in your stomach longer. Along with helping to keep blood sugar in check, it's been shown to lower cholesterol levels.

Insoluble fiber—found in vegetables and grains—comes in two broad categories. Fermentable fiber promotes the growth of "good" bacteria in your colon, and is also thought to inhibit the formation of tumors. Nonfermentable fiber speeds up the transit time of your meals—in one end, out the other.

The long-term benefits of fiber are impressive. Studies show it protects against colon cancer, the third-leading cause of cancer death in the United States. Increased fiber consumption reduces fasting blood-sugar levels in people with type 2 diabetes. It may also reduce blood pressure in people with hypertension.

All that is aside from the benefit you're probably most interested in: weight control. Some research (and a few popular diets) suggests that fiber offers "negative" calories: The more fiber in your diet, the less energy you can metabolize from the other food you eat. That's in addition to the "bulking" effect, which increases both satiation (your stomach feels full faster) and satiety (you're less hungry between meals).

The current guidelines suggest that men eat 38 grams of fiber per day, or 14 grams per 1,000 calories. (It's 25 grams a day for women.) You want to get your fiber from real food, since fiber supplements don't seem to be effective, at least against colon cancer. By contrast, whole grains and legumes are correlated with lower rates of diabetes, heart disease, cancer, and stroke.

Whether that's because of fiber or other nutrients doesn't really matter. There's also the possibility that people who are naturally health- and fitness-conscious eat those foods because they've been told they're supposed to. So of course those foods would then correlate with longevity, disease reduction, a lower body weight, and all the other benefits of healthy, active living. All that really matters here is that they qualify as "whole or minimally processed" for the purpose of Alan's diet plan. It's up to you which ones you want to include, and in what quantities.

Finding Fiber

FOOD	SERVING	FIBER (G)
LEGUMES		
Navy beans, cooked from dried	½ cup	9.6
Split peas, cooked from dried	½ cup	8.1
Lentils, cooked from dried	½ cup	7.8
Kidney beans, canned	½ cup	6.8
CEREALS AND GRAINS		
100% (wheat) bran cereal	½ cup	12.5
Oats	½ cup	8.3
Oat bran, cooked	½ cup	2.9
Quinoa, cooked	½ cup	2.6
Instant oatmeal, cooked	½ cup	2.0
Rice, long-grain brown, cooked	½ cup	1.8

FOOD	SERVING	FIBER (G)
VEGETABLES		
Artichoke hearts, cooked	½ cup	7.2
Spinach, frozen, cooked	½ cup	3.5
Brussels sprouts, frozen, cooked	½ cup	3.2
Winter squash, cooked	1 cup	2.9
Mushrooms, white, cooked from fresh	1 cup	1.7
FRUITS		
Prunes, uncooked	½ cup, pitted	6.2
Guava, fresh	½ cup	4.5
Asian pear	1 small pear	4.4
Raspberries, fresh	½ cup	4.0
Blackberries, fresh	½ cup	3.8
NUTS AND SEEDS		
Almonds	1 ounce (23 kernels)	3.5
Pistachio nuts	1 ounce (49 kernels)	2.9
Pecans	1 ounce (19 halves)	2.7
Peanuts	1 ounce	2.4

Fat Matters

Back in the early '90s, when Alan and I started our careers in the fitness business, it was accepted more or less without question that fat was bad for you. Virginia Tech historian Ann LaBerge, PhD, came up with four reasons why a "low-fat diet" became the answer to almost every health-related question.

> **1.** For most of the 20th century, adults in the United States were told that their adult weight should never change.

Whatever you weigh in your early twenties is what you should *always* weigh. By that standard, nearly every American over 30 needed to lose weight. Since fat has 9 calories per gram versus 4 per gram for carbs and protein, cutting back on fat seemed like the most direct path to weight loss.

2. Diets with a lot of fat and cholesterol, particularly from animal sources, were (somewhat mistakenly) linked to heart disease.

3. The US government took an official stand in the late 1970s, advocating low-fat diets for the prevention of both heart disease and cancer. Every authoritative body—from the World Health Organization to the American Heart Association—went along. Food companies soon figured out they could market complete crap, from cinnamon rolls to ice cream, as heart-healthy, as long as it was low in fat.

4. The media echoed and thus reinforced everything. (Guilty as charged.)

We Americans, in that more innocent time, actually listened to the experts. We believed fat really was bad for us, and that the healthiest diet was the one that contained the least fat. Then came the moment of reckoning.

It was kind of like that scene in *The Godfather,* right after the meeting called by Vito Corleone to make peace with the other Mafia dons. Corleone went into the meeting thinking his chief nemesis was Philip Tattaglia. But Tattaglia, Corleone says to his consigliere on the ride home, "is a pimp." He couldn't possibly have waged the war that Corleone had just ended, a war that cost both dons a son. What follows is one of the greatest lines in movie history: "I didn't know until this day that it was Barzini all along."

Even Corleone, the most powerful of crime lords, a man who later says, "I spent my whole life trying not to be careless," could make a fatal mistake of judgment and perception.

Science, alas, is not cinema. It took a long time to figure out how misguided the war on fat was. The most compelling evidence was cumulative. The obesity rate skyrocketed in the final quarter of the 20th century, even though Americans actually ate less fat as a percentage of total calories consumed. We stopped drinking whole milk, ate less red meat and fewer eggs, used less butter and other fats and oils. But at the same time, we ate more of everything else. A *lot* more. The per capita US food supply increased 15 percent between 1970 and 1994.

Fat, it turns out, was a pimp. It was calories all along.

"Are You a Good Fat, or a Bad Fat?"

Around the time we figured out fats weren't automatically fattening, nutrition experts (and the journalists who quote them) developed a new routine: single out individual types of fat for praise or blame. We used phrases like "heart-healthy" or "artery-clogging" to help consumers understand which fats they should or shouldn't eat. Yet again, we defaulted to black-and-white thinking.

In the "heart-healthy" column were the unsaturated fatty acids. They fall into two broad categories, monounsaturated and polyunsaturated, which merit two of the most entertaining acronyms in all of science: MUFA and PUFA. You could market a line of children's toys with those names and do pretty well with it.

Oleic acid is the most common MUFA. You find it in animal and vegetable foods—olive oil is the usual example—and it makes up close to half of all the fat tissue in your body. MUFAs are universally considered to be a healthy source of energy, provided you don't eat too much. Like any dietary fat, they're easily converted to body fat.

PUFAs are more interesting. When the notion that some fats are good for you first got traction, PUFAs were exhibit A. Two PUFAs are essential fatty acids, which means your body can't make them from other fats. The first is *linoleic acid*, an omega-6 PUFA; the second is *alpha-linolenic acid*, an omega-3.

Linoleic acid is by far the most common PUFA in our diets. An average American guy consumes about 16 grams a day, which is 80 to 90 percent of all the PUFAs in his diet. If he's eating 2,500 calories a day, about 5 percent would be linoleic acid. Almost all of it comes from three sources: soybean, corn, and cottonseed oils, which were virtually unknown in the human diet a century ago.

Meanwhile, we get hardly any omega-3 fats through our diets. If you have even the most basic interest in nutrition, you probably know that the two omega-3 fats found in fish oil—EPA and DHA—have been linked to just about every important aspect of human health. The biggest one is brain development, particularly early and late in life. For a while, fish oil supplements were thought to help prevent cardiovascular disease, although recent evidence doesn't support that idea.

You may have also read about the importance of the ratio of omega-6 to omega-3 fats. This is an article of faith among those who promote the paleo diet, who believe that early humans ate a diet in which the two types of PUFAs were more or less in balance. But in the past few thousand years, with the rise of agriculture and especially the recent introduction of highly processed foods, that ratio has skewed dramatically toward omega-6 fats. What was once a 1-to-1 ratio (or at worst 4-to-1) has become more like 15- or 20-to-1. Since omega-6 fats are linked to inflammation and omega-3s do the opposite, it's an important question. More systemic inflammation could lead to heart disease.

Thus, in theory, changing the ratio of PUFAs should make your heart less FUBAR. But the best, most recent evidence we have suggests you shouldn't bother. Both types of PUFAs are linked to a lower risk of heart disease, and there doesn't seem to be any advantage to balancing them. Instead, the goal should be to get more of each.

To increase the omega-3s in your diet, you could simply eat more fish, which is also a great source of protein. Those of us who don't eat fish very often can take fish oil supplements. Although not directly linked to heart disease prevention, they do lower the level of triglycerides in your blood, which is an indirect way to improve your metabolic health. (High triglycerides are part of metabolic syndrome, along with high blood pressure, high blood sugar, and excess belly fat. The combination is linked to type 2 diabetes.) Alan says three to six capsules a day is a reasonable target. You don't want to go above 10 capsules unless your doctor recommends it; at that dose, you would get 3 grams of EPA and DHA, which could interfere with blood clotting.

The best way to get more omega-6 fats is to eat more nuts. To Alan, nuts may be the strongest argument against the importance of balancing the two types of PUFAs. That's because nuts are outrageously unbalanced—almonds have more than 2,000 times as much omega-6 as omega-3—and yet they're associated with a long list of health benefits. People who eat the most nuts tend to be the leanest, with the lowest risk of diabetes, respiratory problems, and cardiovascular disease.

So, to review:

▶ MUFAs are good for you.

▶ PUFAs are good for you.

▶ There's no good reason to worry about the ratio of omega-6 to omega-3 PUFAs in your diet.

But there must be some types of fat that are bad for you. Your parents and teachers and doctors and scientists couldn't have been *entirely* wrong. Could they?

Saturation Coverage

If you Google "artery clogging," almost all the links will lead you to articles about trans fats. These are fatty acids that have been changed from liquid vegetable oil to a solid fat through a process called hydrogenation. The history of hydrogenation goes back to the early 1900s, when Procter & Gamble fought the Brown Company for the patent rights. P&G was founded in 1837 to manufacture soap and candles. They branched out into the lard business in the late 1800s, and would eventually use hydrogenation to make Crisco shortening. (One of its early names was Cryst, short for "crystallized cottonseed oil." The company decided against it for obvious religious reasons.) Crisco was cheaper and more stable than lard or butter, and thus gave baked goods a longer shelf life. But P&G's original use for hydrogenation was to make soap. Thus, if you want to eat a diet that's truly "clean," it doesn't get any cleaner than hydrogenated vegetable oil.

In the 1950s and '60s, as the experts beat the drum against saturated fats, another product of hydrogenation, margarine, became a popular alternative to butter. We now know that was a terrible mistake; trans fats produced by hydrogenation are strongly linked to heart disease.

What was wrong with butter? Every kid who's taken a nutrition class in school can tell you butter is loaded with "artery-clogging" saturated fat. I would guess that every journalist who's written about nutrition in the past two decades has used that phrase in reference to the fats found in meat, eggs, dairy, and a handful of plant foods, like palm and coconut oils.

Saturated fats do indeed raise your cholesterol levels, but by itself that doesn't mean you're at higher risk of heart disease. The more diligently scientists looked at saturated fats, the less evidence of harm they found. There seems to be some small benefit to replacing saturated fats with PUFAs (a 2 to 3 percent reduction in cardiovascular disease risk), but absolutely no benefit to replacing saturated fats with carbohydrates, which was the standard advice for decades. In fact, that may actually be *worse* for your health.

So where does that leave us?

The US government's current recommendation is to get 20 to 35 percent of your total calories from fat, which Alan says is "reasonable, safe, and flexible, and one of the few things I feel the government got right." It's easily enough fat for basic biological functions, like transporting fat-soluble vitamins (A, D, E, and K), manufacturing hormones and other chemical messengers, and providing structural integrity to cells. Moreover, fat is a perfectly fine source of energy, and gives our food texture and flavor. In combination with protein, fat helps us feel satisfied after a meal.

In Alan's diet plan, you'll shoot for 0.4 to 0.7 gram of fat per pound of target body weight. So if your target is 180 pounds, your diet will include 72 to 126 grams of fat per day. The lower end is for those who prefer a lower-fat diet, for whatever reasons; the higher end is for those who need or prefer a lower-carb diet.

You'll see all of Alan's recommended food choices in Part Two. His overarching advice about fat will sound familiar by now: Eat a variety of whole and minimally processed foods. In a typical day that might include a handful of walnuts, half an avocado, some fats and oils used for cooking or to dress a salad, and some incidental fat in eggs, a steak, or a nice salmon fillet. Maybe you'll have a small dessert or piece of chocolate with the 10 percent of calories that don't come from whole or minimally processed sources.

Two things you don't want to do:

1. Go out of your way to get more fat in your diet, based on the misguided idea that certain fats like coconut oil or butter from grass-fed cows have superpowers.

2. Load up on one type of fat, like omega-3 PUFAs, instead of getting a variety of them from all categories—saturated, monounsaturated, and polyunsaturated.

Micronutrients Matter

You remember, of course, that there are three macronutrients—protein, carbohydrate, and fat—and you understand why each is important. Also known as *energy nutrients,* you need a lot of them to survive. (Hence, the "macro" part.) Because we have to eat them in large, measurable quantities, they can be studied in a manageable way. Not so with micronutrients, aka vitamins and minerals. The World Health Organization describes them as "'magic wands' that enable the body to produce enzymes, hormones, and other substances essential for proper growth and development." But like lots of allegedly magical things, they come in minuscule amounts—too small to see, and difficult to measure.

History's best-known micronutrient deficiencies include scurvy (lack of vitamin C; it was rectified with the addition of citrus fruit to sailors' rations), beriberi (lack of vitamin B_1, aka thiamin; it still occurs in prisons and refugee camps in the developing world), and rickets (lack of vitamin D and/or calcium; it still affects children in developing countries).

Today iron deficiency is the most common and widespread in the world; it cuts across both geographic and socioeconomic boundaries. In the United States it's the leading cause of anemia. Particularly at risk are young children (3 to 6 months old), adolescent girls, and pregnant women. Women runners are also at higher risk, especially those who are vegetarians.

If you proudly refer to yourself as a "meathead," linking your passion for lifting with your love of a good steak, there's virtually no chance you'll have to worry about an iron deficiency. But there are other deficiency risks to healthy, athletic guys. Take bodybuilders, for example. When my friend Susan Kleiner, PhD, studied the diets of competitive physique athletes, she found that the men got just 46 percent of the Recommended Dietary Allowance for vitamin D, thanks to bodybuilders' traditional milk phobia during contest prep. (They still beat the women in the study by 46 percent. That's right: The female bodybuilders got *zero percent* of the RDA for vitamin D.)

Another way to self-inflict a deficiency is to follow a popular diet to the letter. One recent review looked at four of those diets.

- ▶ Best Life, which advocates a Mediterranean-style diet

- ▶ Atkins for Life, which is low-carb

- ▶ DASH, a low-fat diet recommended for patients with high blood pressure

- ▶ South Beach, a low-carb diet that's considered a kinder, gentler take on Atkins, with much less saturated fat

The meal plans average about 1,750 daily calories, which is ambitious but shouldn't put anyone in the starvation zone. But all were deficient in multiple micronutrients. All four, for example, offer 11 percent or less of the RDA for chromium, which is important for glucose metabolism. They're also low in vitamins D and E, as well as iodine, a deficiency in which is the leading cause of brain damage in the developing world. (In the United States we damage our brains in more robust ways, by playing contact sports and listening to AM radio.)

We don't want to overstate the dangers of these diets, since we don't know of any documented cases of serious harm. For one thing, it's unlikely anyone can follow the strictest version of any diet for more than a few weeks at a time. The big point is this: The more extreme and restrictive your diet, the more likely it is you'll self-inflict a deficiency. (Paradoxically, the same is true for the sloppiest, least-restrictive diets. Some of the most overweight people also have severe micronutrient deficiencies.)

So should you take a "just in case" multivitamin? That's a surprisingly complicated question. Most vitamin research can be summed up with one word: "meh," followed by dozens of references. The most we can say is that a basic, inexpensive multi, taken daily, can't hurt, and might help in some minor way. Alan recommends two brands: Kirkland and Nature Made. Both have USP verification, which ensures label accuracy, purity, and potency, and that it will dissolve in your stomach and be properly absorbed.

Even with a multi, you might not get enough vitamin D and magnesium. Magnesium tends to be underdosed in multis because the full RDA of 400 milligrams per day for adult men would require a pill the size of a horse suppository. About half the US population is considered deficient, a consequence of eating too many refined grains and too few nuts, fruits, and vegetables. Since magnesium is involved in hundreds of metabolic processes, including the use of fat for energy, a supplemental boost could be useful.

With vitamin D, the amounts you find in supplements are based on the minimum to prevent rickets. And they aren't necessarily the most useful form of the vitamin. Alan and many other nutritionists think guys should at least consider supplementing with 1,000 to 2,000 IU of vitamin D_3—the potential benefits include stronger bones and better immune-system function. But before you supplement, keep in mind that simply stepping outside for a few minutes on a sunny day can generate 10 times the amount of vitamin D you'd get from a pill.

Here's Alan's biggest point about micronutrients: "A poor diet with a multivitamin is still a poor diet." Which brings us to perhaps the most polarizing question a guy can ask in the early 21st century: "WTF is a *good* diet?"

Just about every popular weight loss plan in recent years is based on eliminating something that most of us grew up eating. Vegans avoid meat, fish, eggs, and dairy. The paleo diet goes after grains, legumes, and sometimes even potatoes. Atkins-type low-carb diets go even further, proscribing fruits and nuts in the early stages. The result, as noted earlier, is that a lot of important vitamins and minerals are left off the menu.

Alan's model diet dusts off and reboots the old-fashioned idea of food groups. He came up with six.

- ▶ **Meat and other protein-rich foods.** These include animal flesh, eggs, and protein powder.

- ▶ **Fat-rich foods.** Here you have nuts and seeds, any type of oil used for dressing a salad or cooking, butter and nut butters, olives, and avocados.

- ▶ **Fibrous vegetables.** Leafy greens, broccoli and cauliflower, asparagus . . . if your mother once made dessert contingent on eating something specific, it probably falls into this category.

- ▶ **Starchy foods.** You remember these from way back in the carbohydrate section. They include grains, legumes (beans and peas), and tubers (potatoes and other root vegetables).

- ▶ **Milk and other dairy products.** Basically, milk, yogurt, and cheese. There are obvious crossovers with protein- and fat-rich foods, which we'll get into in more detail in Part Two.

- ▶ **Fruits.** You want to eat whole, fresh fruit. Juices are okay when there's no other choice (as long as they're 100 percent fruit), but processing always takes something away, and you never know how much of the nutritional value is lost.

Alan lists them in this order for the sake of his easy-to-remember mnemonic device: "Meg's fabulous figure stopped missing fries." The first two letters of each word are also the first two letters of each food group.

ALAN EXPLAINS WHY PERSONAL PREFERENCE MATTERS

YOU CHOOSE, YOU LOSE

You want to know something that bugs the hell out of me? Diets that tell you explicitly which foods are "allowed" and which are "prohibited." Most of the foods on the no-fry list will be the usual crap, like doughnuts and chips and non-diet sodas. But some will be perfectly tolerable and nutritious. The more insidious problem is that some of those tolerable and nutritious foods will be among your favorites. For the majority of us, these no-no's are nonsensical.

Take the banning of grains, for example. It started out as a hallmark of the paleo diet, but since then it has become kind of a faith system, spawning best-selling books that make outrageous, unsupportable claims about how just one grain—wheat—has sabotaged the health of a generation of innocent Americans.

The reason for the antigrain hysteria is gluten, which a very small percentage of us can't tolerate in our diets. Celiac disease is a gluten-triggered autoimmune reaction within the small intestine, and if you're among the nearly 1 percent of Americans who have it, you should avoid wheat and other gluten-containing grains at all costs.

In addition, the Celiac Disease Center at Columbia University estimates about half a percent of Americans have non-celiac gluten sensitivity, aka gluten intolerance, which has similar symptoms but doesn't yet have a clear set of diagnostic criteria.

So that's roughly 1.5 percent of Americans. With a population north of 300 million, that's a lot of people—probably 4 to 5 million—who should avoid gluten. But that still leaves more than 95 percent of Americans who don't have that problem, and certainly don't have a medical reason to avoid all grains, most of which have no gluten whatsoever, as you can see in this chart.

GLUTEN-CONTAINING GRAINS	GLUTEN-FREE GRAINS
Wheat, including varieties like spelt, kamut, farro, and durum; and products like bulgur and semolina	Amaranth
Barley	Buckwheat
Rye	Corn
Triticale	Job's Tears (or Hato Mugi)
	Millet
	Montina (Indian ricegrass)
Oats*	Oats*
	Quinoa
	Rice
	Sorghum
	Teff
	Wild rice

*Oats are gluten-free, but can sometimes be contaminated with wheat during growing or processing. Several companies—Bob's Red Mill, Cream Hill Estates, GF Harvest (formerly Gluten Free Oats), and Avena Foods (Only Oats)—offer uncontaminated oats.

I'll return to the paleo diet shortly. First, though, let's talk about what may be the most important element of every successful diet, and the one that's most neglected.

WHY PERSONAL PREFERENCE MATTERS

Suppose I came to you with this proposition: *The best diet for long-term adherence is the one that's based on foods you hate.* I'll grant that you could lose a lot of weight with that diet, since you'd rather starve than eat foods you find repellent. But it would obviously be the worst diet for adherence. You'd never be able to stick with it.

Change one word, though, and it makes all kinds of sense: *The best diet for long-term adherence is the one that's based on foods you love.*

I've said many times, in many places, and in many ways that honoring personal preference is the most overlooked and underutilized tool for long-term success in a weight loss plan. This isn't just a special intuition of mine. We have solid science to back it up.

Back in 2005, a team at Tufts Medical Center studied four diets that were popular at the time: Ornish (restricts fat), Zone (balances macronutrients), Weight Watchers (restricts calories), and Atkins (restricts carbs). After 1 year, the average guy in the study had lost just over 7 pounds, which was 3.1 percent of his starting weight. The average woman had lost just over 5 pounds, or 2.5 percent of her initial size. For weight loss, there was no statistical difference between diets; they were all equally mediocre.

There was, however, a difference in dropout rates: About 50 percent of the people assigned to the two most restrictive diets—Ornish and Atkins—bailed before the 12 months were up, compared with 35 percent for Zone and Weight Watchers, which are more flexible.

But that's not why the study is important.

In each diet group, about a quarter of the participants lost more than 5 percent of their starting weight, and about 10 percent lost more than 10 percent. A guy in that latter group who started the diet on January 1 at 220 pounds would be under 200 on December 31.

Just one factor separated the big losers from the mere finishers: adherence. Those who stayed closest to their assigned plan lost the most weight. The effect was the same across all four diets.

It's not an isolated finding. In study after study, researchers find that diets work about equally well. The difference is typically just a few pounds. What matters, consistently, is whether people can stick closely enough to their assigned diets to see results.

Which leads me to one of my wackier ideas. Suppose I told you to list your 20 favorite foods and then said, "That's your diet." Let's call it the Personal Favorites Diet. You eat those things, and only those things. Each person's diet would be wildly different, but you know you'd look forward to every meal.

I know what you're thinking: "What if all 20 of my foods are desserts?" You think it would fail. So let's turn it around. Suppose I gave you a list of 20 "superfoods" that I say are the cleanest, most nutritious foods on the planet—just packed with pure, wholesome nutrition. But you detest almost all the foods on my list. Knowing that adherence is the key to a successful diet, which diet do you think would work better?

My guess is that you'd have no chance on Alan's superfoods diet. You wouldn't be able to stick to it for more than a week or two. But that Personal Favorites Diet? You'd certainly stick to it. And if we found a way for that diet to include fewer calories than you eat now, you'd even lose weight.

This is all just a thought experiment, of course. I'd never gamble with your health by putting you on a diet that might be 100 percent processed food. That's why the Lean Muscle Plan is 80 percent (say it with me) whole and minimally processed foods you like, 10 percent (say it with me again) whole and minimally processed foods you don't necessarily hate, and 10 percent pure, junky goodness.

TOLERANCE: THE FINAL PIECE OF THE PUZZLE

I started this by telling you what drives me nuts about popular diets. I hate when gurus decide that foods *some* people can't tolerate should be avoided by *everybody*. To show you how logically incoherent this is, let's look at the eight major food allergens, as identified by the Food Allergen Labeling and Consumer Protection Act of 2004.

- Milk
- Eggs
- Fish (e.g., bass, flounder, cod)
- Crustacean shellfish (e.g., crab, lobster, shrimp)
- Tree nuts (e.g., almonds, walnuts, pecans)
- Peanuts
- Wheat
- Soybeans

Altogether, about 2.7 percent of Americans have been diagnosed with an allergy to one or more of the eight. All these foods are dangerous to a small percentage of us. But you won't find a popular diet that tells you not to eat any of them. They all pick and choose, for different reasons. The paleo diet, for example, tells you not to eat four of the eight—milk, peanuts, wheat, and soybeans—but allows virtually unlimited amounts of the others. The reason, as most of you know, is that those foods weren't common in the diets of our ancestors in the Paleolithic era, or the Stone Age, which lasted until the rise of agriculture about 10,000 years ago.

Let's look at just one of those foods: milk.

Dairy foods are nutritional powerhouses. They're the number-one source of calcium, vitamin D, phosphorus, and potassium in Americans' diets. All those nutrients are crucial for the strength and health of your bones. Dairy is also an important source of protein.

It's true that many people can't digest lactose, the sugar in milk, beyond early childhood. Worldwide, about 65 percent of humans are lactose intolerant; for people of East Asian descent, it's more than 90 percent. But the majority of Americans, whose ancestors came from Europe, have no problem with lactose. Even among those who are diagnosed with lactose intolerance, most can enjoy the equivalent of one cup of milk without discomfort, especially when the milk is consumed with other foods. So why would you try to convince anyone who tolerates dairy to avoid it entirely?

To me, it doesn't make any sense at all.

—AA

CHAPTER 3:

WHAT MAKES A WORKOUT WORK

F IT'S NOT CLEAR ALREADY, I should come clean about something: I'm probably older than you. Possibly a *lot* older. I was born in 1957 and started working out around 1970, when my older brother brought home our first weight set from Sears. We put the weights in our basement and taught ourselves to lift. That's how I became an expert on not getting results.

The late '50s and early '60s were the height of the baby boom and the lowest point of interest in health, nutrition, and exercise. I was bottle-fed because if an American corporation made it, it just had to be better than what you could get from any ol' boob. Both my parents and most of our neighbors smoked. Why wouldn't they? Cigarette ads were everywhere; to this day I can recall jingles and slogans for at least a half-dozen brands, and back then I didn't know of any place on earth where smoking wasn't allowed. Fast food was a rare treat, but when we went to McDonald's, we went all-in. I remember dipping my french fries into my vanilla milk shake and not thinking that was at all weird.

Imagine the dearth of information about training in those days. This wasn't just pre-Internet—it was pre–cable TV and VCRs. Bookstores were maybe a quarter the size of your local Barnes & Noble. If I knew workout books or muscle magazines existed, I somehow blocked it from memory. We didn't even have broscience. Instead we had Charles Atlas ads in the backs of comic books. The premise of the ads was that you could start off as a skinny weakling (which, alas, I was), go work out for a while, and come back so muscular and intimidating that you could drive a bully off with a single punch.

Since the ads didn't tell us how to train, or how long it would take (beyond the deliberately ambiguous "later"), we just assumed size and strength were universally attainable. That is, we thought any of us could not only make ourselves bigger and stronger than we were at the moment, we could also be objectively *big* and *strong,* with muscles that would make us intimidating to our rivals, good at sports, popular with our peers, and of course irresistible to the girls. This magical idea disregarded not only the limitations imposed by genetics, but also the importance of diet and training methods. All it took, we thought, was desire.

Which, it turns out, wasn't nearly enough. I learned the hard way that all those other things—diet, genetics, and how you train—really do matter. We talked about diet in Chapter 2, and we'll talk about genetics in Chapter 4. Here we'll take a deep dive into the basic principles behind successful workouts.

Movements, Not Muscles

The simplest and most intuitive way to plan your workout is to build it around muscles. You care about your biceps and abs and pecs, so of course you fill your time in the weight room with exercises that target the muscles you want to make big and ripply. Those exercises give you immediate feedback: You feel them work the muscles directly when you do a biceps curl or an ab crunch or a chest fly. Your upper body is getting bigger and veinier with every set. What a specimen you'll soon become!

But what happens when you don't become that specimen—assuming you still want to train when results don't come quickly or easily? In my experience, three reactions are typical.

▶ You stick with your original plan for the rest of your life, waiting for it to work.

▶ Your random workouts become more random. You add more exercises for the same muscles that weren't growing with the old exercises.

▶ You go guru shopping, jumping from one well-marketed training system to the next. Sometimes the new system feels like it's working for a month or two, but when the results slow down you get bored and move on.

I think there's a much better way to get results, to get them sooner, and to get them more consistently over time. It's based on a question I never thought to ask when I was 13, or 23, or even 33. By the time it finally dawned on me, I'd been writing about fitness for years and had a couple of personal-training certifications on my résumé. Here's the question: What is your body supposed to do?

Put another way: What are your muscles for? Just by asking the question you know the answer isn't crunches, curls, calf raises, and leg extensions. Different experts will offer different answers, but it's hard to go wrong with these basic human movements.

Walking

Humans probably separated from the great apes at least 5 million years ago. The australopithecines, the first humanlike species, are thought to have lived in trees but also to have walked upright. Over millions of years, climbing became less important while walking long distances in search of food became a bigger part of the survival strategy. Legs got longer and arms got shorter as humans evolved. Eventually humans walked to, and settled in, every habitable place on the planet.

But unless you're Frodo Baggins, schlepping the One Ring up Mount Doom with the fate of humankind on your shoulders, walking is easy. It's not exercise so much as a way to get from one room to another. Nobody goes into the gym thinking, "My goal is to look like a walker!"

Running and Jumping

On the other hand, most of us would love to look in the mirror and see an Olympic sprinter or long jumper looking back. All-out running and max-distance jumping are functions of muscle power, the ability to produce force as quickly as possible. Power, though, is highly correlated with strength—the ability to express maximum force, regardless of speed. And strength, however imperfectly, is correlated with muscle size. Thus, pure-power athletes like 100-meter sprinters carry the most muscle mass they can pack on before it begins to slow them down.

You can see why early humans needed to sprint from time to time. It would have been important for hunting and to avoid being hunted. The ability to jump was crucial for similarly obvious reasons. That's why our body's biggest, strongest muscles—glutes, hamstrings, quadriceps—are the ones that power sprints and jumps.

That said, the strength of those muscles is relative. The beasts hunting us were quite a bit faster, and many of them could jump a lot farther. Our survival depended, in part, on being able to construct shelter against both weather and hungry predators. That was made possible by some of the unique ways we use our upper-body muscles.

Pushing and Pulling, and Lifting and Carrying

Humans aren't the only animals who can manipulate their environment. Beavers can change the course of rivers; prairie dogs create underground suburbs; and ants build fantastically complicated habitats, with a level of unforced cooperation that the most ruthless dictator can only dream about. Humans' abilities to build or destroy are at a completely different level, thanks to our unprecedented brainpower. But all the cleverness of the first human architects and engineers would have been useless without the ability to push some things out of their way, pull other things to where they wanted them, and, perhaps most important of all, lift the things they found in one place—building materials, supplies, food, children, injured comrades—and carry them to another place.

Picture this: You just killed a hundred-pound antelope. You're a mile from home, and there's no one nearby to help with the load. So you pull the antelope into position, squat down, and grab it with both hands. It takes you a couple tries, but eventually you manage to sling it over your shoulders. You stand up and shift it across your back so the weight is evenly distributed. That was pretty tough. But the long walk home is a far bigger challenge—shifting terrain, changes in elevation, obstacles you have to go over or around.

By the time you get there, just about every muscle in your body feels tired and sore, if not thrashed. Your calves, for example, are on fire, having just performed hundreds of repetitions with your body weight plus the weight of the dead animal. Even some muscles that *didn't* move, like those in your back and shoulders, are equally exhausted from the strain of holding the carcass in place and keeping you upright.

Again, we're hardly the only species that picks things up and moves them around. African termites create mounds as tall as we are, which is all the more impressive when you realize they use their own excrement for building material. What definitively sets us apart is a skill that's uniquely human, involving a technically complex coordination of the upper and lower body.

Throwing

We humans are a ridiculously vulnerable species, especially from the front. We have long necks and exposed throats. We don't have any armor protecting our viscera, and only a small rib cage guarding our heart and lungs. Even worse, our nuts are *right there,* begging to be bludgeoned.

Our ability to throw allowed us to play offense long enough and skillfully enough to rise to the top of the food chain. Of all evolutionary adaptations, it ranks second in importance to walking upright. But it's not just throwing in isolation. What matters are all the ways our bodies changed to accommodate our throws.

The earliest humans, the ones closest to apes, had shoulders that were better suited to hanging from trees. But over time the collarbones got longer, the shoulder complex got wider, the torso lengthened, and the hips and waist grew streamlined. Not only did these changes create the V shape that today marks us as sexy beasts, it left us with upper arms hanging straight down from joints that permit maximum range of motion. The combination of free-moving shoulders, narrow hips, and a flexible waist, all of which emerged about 2 million years ago, gave us the ability to throw with both force and precision.

Today we have pitchers who can throw a baseball 100 miles per hour and make it look as easy as you or me playing catch. Quarterbacks can sling a football 70 yards and hit a moving target. The world record in the javelin throw is over 300 feet. But long before we invented sports to make use of this unique ability, we used it for our survival. Without claws or fangs, the ability to whip a rock could have been a difference-maker on offense or defense. Our ancestors eventually graduated to ballistic weapons. The oldest spears found by archaeologists are about 400,000 years old, but no one thinks those were the first spears used. It wouldn't have taken more than a million years to figure out the benefits of throwing a pointed stick.

As with walking, none of us goes into the gym with dreams of looking like a pitcher. It's not throwing itself that you want to exploit so much as the physical adaptations and complex, coordinated movements that made throwing possible. And it *is* complex stuff. I've never seen a kid figure out how to throw without being taught. Inevitably, they stride forward with the wrong leg, or try to throw without striding at all. It's the same with just about any other sport-specific activity that involves a long step forward and some kind of rotation of the upper torso.

In all these actions, whether you're hitting or throwing, the outcome depends on the amount of force you can generate through your lower body, and how well you can channel that force through your torso. Even when you're kicking a ball, you begin with one leg striding forward to generate force through the other leg.

The big point is this: Legs and arms simply don't work in isolation. So why do we train them that way?

The Best Exercises for Size and Strength

To watch the average guy in the average gym go through a workout, you would never guess the human body was meant to do any of the things I just described. Machines like the leg press and leg extension are used in place of the squat, the exercise that comes closest to jumping. (See "The Original Sin of Bodybuilding," later in this chapter, for more on machines.) Pulling exercises, like rows and lat pulldowns, are done while seated, which disassociates the top half of the body from the bottom. And when most people do exercises for their abdominal muscles, they usually do some variation on the crunch. If you were *trying* to design an exercise to perfectly divorce muscles from their function, it would be hard to beat that one.

But when the goal is to build a workout around fundamental human movements, we end up with the following.

Primary Movement Patterns

These four exercise categories do the heavy lifting in the Lean Muscle Plan.

Squat

I don't want to say any single exercise is more important than any other. But the squat has the most potential to build mass, since it uses virtually all your lower-body muscles. Moreover, it's the one exercise that researchers have consistently correlated with sports performance. Improve your strength in the squat and you'll almost certainly increase your speed and the height of your jumps.

Most of us think of the squat as something you do with a barbell on the back of your shoulders, the way powerlifters do it. That's a great exercise for advanced lifters. The rest of us need some intermediate steps to get there. The basic movement is easy and natural for small children (especially the smallest children, who don't yet have bony kneecaps) but complicated for adults, since you have to coordinate actions at the hip, knee, and ankle joints, along with stability in the core muscles to keep your spine in a safe position. (You'll find much, much more on squats—and all the other exercises—in Part Three.)

Deadlift

The deadlift may be the most immediately useful exercise. For a guy, the ability to lift something heavy up off the floor comes into play more often than any other feat of everyday strength. If nothing else, it's a great way to help a friend or impress a stranger—especially when the stranger happens to be cute, single, new to the area, and in need of someone to help carry a couch up the stairs.

The basic movement pattern is simple enough: Start with your hips in a hinged position, and straighten them as you lift an object off the floor, while keeping your lower back stable. That's why the deadlift and its variations work so well to build size and strength in rear-body muscles. As a skinny kid growing up, this exercise would've helped me avoid the dreaded "sideways syndrome"—I might look fit from the front or back, but if I turned to the side, I was so narrow I was practically invisible.

Push and Pull

Show me a guy who created his own workout program and I'll show you someone who's probably doing more pushing exercises—the ones that work the chest, shoulders, and triceps—than pulling. Pulls work the lats (the fan-shaped muscles on the sides of your torso), trapezius (the diamond-shaped muscle that runs from the bottom of the neck, out to both shoulder blades, and down to the middle of the back), rear deltoids (the back part of the muscle that covers your shoulder joints), and biceps.

We all understand why we do more pushes than pulls: We want to look in the mirror and see those pecs and delts. But remember what I wrote in Chapter 1: Women judge your physique, and by extension your reproductive suitability, by the proportion of your shoulders to your waist. You create that V shape primarily with pulling exercises, like chinups and rows. Those exercises widen and thicken your upper torso.

That's not to say the pushing exercises—pushups, bench presses, shoulder presses—aren't important. They certainly are. But you'll go a lot further with balanced development of strength and size than you will by trying to accelerate the growth of one set of muscles at the expense of another.

This is especially important when the goal is to build bigger arms. Most of us instinctively prioritize arm development without stopping to ask why our biceps, triceps, and forearms would grow out of proportion to the chest, shoulders, and upper-back muscles—the ones they're designed to work with. In fact, your arm muscles will grow pretty well without *any* exercises designed to target them. That's because presses, rows, and chinups allow you to work with much heavier weights than you can use for curls or triceps extensions. The big upper-body muscles are the prime movers in those exercises, but you can't do them without assistance from your arms. Thus, your arms will develop size and strength in proportion to the growth of your chest, shoulders, and upper back.

My point isn't to argue that arm exercises have no place in your training; they're a minor part of the Lean Muscle Plan, and you have the option to do more on your own. You just have to understand where their place is relative to the exercises that use bigger muscles in more useful movements.

Complementary Movement Patterns

You could put together an outstanding workout with variations on the four primary movements—squat, deadlift, push, pull—and little else. You would work all your body's major muscles and, depending on the time and effort you put in, end up with a better-looking physique than a guy who did dozens of exercises designed to hit one muscle at a time.

Of course, you'd have to know what you're doing, or follow a program designed by someone who has that knowledge. For example, you'd want to rotate through the best variations for your goals, both to keep the workouts fresh and to avoid the kind of joint stress that comes from repeating the exact same movements in the exact same way. You'd also need to slot the exercises into a program in which you work toward different goals at different times, starting with lighter weights and higher workout volume—more sets and reps—and working your way toward heavier weights with fewer sets and reps. Then, when you feel you've gotten all you can out of that sequence, you'd start over again with a slightly different configuration but the same basic goal: to end up with more muscle, less fat, greater strength, and improved skill as a lifter.

But while it would work, it still wouldn't be an ideal program. It's missing three important exercise categories.

Split Stance

Walking, running, climbing, throwing—all are done with one leg in front of or higher than the other. Even jumps often take off from one leg, rather than both. Thus, each leg needs the strength to propel your body weight, as well as the balance to support it when the other leg is off the ground.

Lunges and stepups are great exercises on their own for the usual reasons. They work all your lower-body muscles, and develop strength in useful movement patterns. They also provide what you could call "just in case" strength. Muscles are naturally weaker near the end of their range of motion. Split-stance exercises train your muscles to work from those lengthened positions. I'm not saying they prevent injuries—I don't know of any research showing cause and effect—but they certainly work muscles that might otherwise be undertrained. And that's never a bad outcome.

Carry

If the ability to lift and carry is a crucial evolutionary trait, then it stands to reason that there's a benefit to training your body to carry heavier things. Indeed, research on the farmer's walk—an exercise in which you carry something heavy in each of your hands—shows that the abdominal muscles fire repeatedly to keep your body stabilized. In addition, the act of lifting the objects off the ground hits the same back muscles you use in the deadlift.

There are certainly more *direct* ways to work abdominal muscles, as you'll see in a moment. For that matter, I don't think muscle activation is the main selling point of carries. It's that they're a pretty good workout all by themselves. A few sets of carries leave you gasping for breath and sweating like an air-conditioning repairman in August. The more effort you put in, the bigger the postworkout metabolic boost you should get over the following hours, when your systems are running faster than normal to help your body recover.

And to tell you the truth, I'm not even sure that's the best reason to do them. I like them because they present a systemic challenge. They test your posture, balance, endurance, and grip strength, as well as your body's overall ability to do difficult things—one of the most important of which is to lift and carry heavy objects.

Core-Stability Exercises

Heavy carries are about as far from traditional core-training exercises as you'll get. If nothing else, they show that every exercise, done correctly, works your core one way or another. Still, I think it makes sense to train your core muscles directly, which is why I wrote an entire book about it.

In *The New Rules of Lifting for Abs,* Alwyn Cosgrove and I argue that the core includes all the muscles that act on the lower back, pelvis, and hip joints. Which, yes, is a pretty massive collection of contractile tissue. It includes:

- ▶ Abdominals

- ▶ Lower-back muscles

- ▶ Hip flexors (the ones that lift your legs out in front of you)

- ▶ Hip extensors (the glutes and hamstrings, which straighten your hips when you're bent forward)

And your lats, we wrote, may be the most important core muscles that you never thought of as part of the core. The lats' main gig is to pull your arms in toward your torso. That's why you target them with exercises like rows and pulldowns. But the muscles originate from multiple places, including a thick sheet of connective tissue in your lower back called the sacrolumbar fascia, which extends all the way down to your tailbone. Those tissues have to contract to help stabilize your lower back when you lift something heavy off the floor. To contract them, you pull your shoulders down and tighten up your lat muscles. You don't necessarily need to think about it for it to happen; an experienced lifter will do this automatically. If you don't activate that protective mechanism, you leave your lower back more vulnerable to injury while losing much of the strength you'd otherwise be able to generate.

The role of the core muscles—when they're acting as core muscles—is to stabilize the middle of your body and protect your spine while other muscles are generating force. In the Lean Muscle Plan you'll do three types of core-training exercises.

Stability: You're probably familiar with planks and side planks. These basic exercises require you to stabilize your core muscles for a prescribed amount of time. As soon as you meet the thresholds described in Part Three, you'll move on to more advanced and challenging variations.

Dynamic stability: In these exercises you train your core muscles for the function I just described—stabilizing your lower back while other muscles are in motion. In some of them your arms move out away from your body, challenging your core to make sure your lower back doesn't sink into a deeper arch. In others your legs move up toward your chest. The challenge is to keep your back from flattening out of its natural position. Then there are rotational challenges, in which you work to keep your spine from twisting while you turn your shoulders.

Strength and hypertrophy: The goal of stability and dynamic-stability exercises is to improve core endurance—holding your lower back and pelvis in a safe position. Core strength is a different quality. In theory, it should be a component of any program that aims to build total-body strength in pursuit of a leaner, more muscular, and more athletic body.

But it's trickier to accomplish. The rectus abdominis, the "six-pack" muscle, isn't like your biceps or hamstrings. It doesn't need to be trained through a range of motion, by forcing it to shorten and lengthen and then shorten again, as you would during a crunch. There aren't many actions in sports or everyday life that include a forward bend at the waist against some kind of resistance. It would come into play in combat sports, but I can't really think of anything else. Otherwise, the abdominal muscles are there to support the muscles above, below, and behind them in all the actions I've already described—pulling, pushing, throwing, lifting and carrying, running and jumping, and climbing.

Furthermore, there's no point in trying to isolate individual or small groups of core muscles; not only is it physiologically impossible, it's functionally pointless. You need them to work together. That's what we want to accomplish with the strength exercises: challenge the core muscles to get stronger while using them in some approximation of natural movement patterns.

Accessory Movements

I should note here that, despite the official-sounding terms, these categories are arbitrary. They're based on my understanding of exercise science and practice, which is hardly encyclopedic. (My undergrad degree is in journalism, and I went to grad school for creative writing.) But just because they aren't written on stone tablets doesn't mean they're random. I spent countless hours doing the exercises in this category—the biceps curls, triceps extensions, shoulder exercises, and calf raises—through many years of semiproductive training. But the more I learn about this subject and the longer I write about it, the less important these exercises seem. I never come across compelling reasons to waste a lot of time and energy targeting your body's smaller muscles.

The peak of my accessory-movement obsession came in the early 1990s, shortly after I went to work for *Men's Fitness* magazine. It was owned by Weider Publications, which also published *Muscle & Fitness* and *Flex*. I read in one of those magazines that Joe Weider, founder and publisher, could still curl 90 pounds well into middle age. Based on that ridiculous (and possibly untrue) anecdote, I decided that being able to curl 90 pounds was an important benchmark of total-body strength, and set out to achieve it. I'm pretty sure I managed a couple of reps—probably with atrocious form—and felt momentarily good about myself. Even better, my upper-arm girth exceeded 15 inches for the first (and only) time in my life.

So, yes, spending a lot of time and effort on arm exercises will give you bigger arms. But in my case, those bigger arms came with bigger everything, thanks to indiscriminate eating and a sedentary job. I weighed at least 10 pounds more than I do now. When I look at pictures of myself from those years, I see a soft-looking guy with no obvious muscular development. I'd been working out for more than 20 years by then, and the only person who thought I looked like a lifter was me.

Which is not to say that arm exercises were to blame. It was my fault for spending too much time on them and too little time on everything else, and for eating like a moron. (*Especially* for eating like a moron.) Biceps curls actually have a long, distinguished history. Old-time weightlifters and strongmen did them, and for a while the curl was used in powerlifting competitions. In the first half of my career as a fitness writer, every workout article included arm exercises. It never occurred to me *not* to include them.

Then my coauthors and I stopped using them. Partly it was because the magazine format became more condensed. It's hard to justify putting arm exercises into a total-body workout when you have space for just five or six movements. But it wasn't just because magazines changed. We stopped using them in books as well, figuring that our readers had limited time to accomplish their often ambitious goals.

You would think my sensible, well-intentioned arguments against time-wasting arm exercises would be convincing. Alas, I've seen no evidence of that. If anything, regular guys in gyms seemed to be more focused on them than ever before. At least once a week I'll see a guy walk into the weight room, go straight to the dumbbell rack, and run through every arm exercise he can think of. Some of them eventually move on to presses and rows. But some don't. Guys who are clearly beginners, by appearance and performance, will spend an entire workout on arm exercises. I'll be blunt: The workouts I see today are the most idiotic I've ever seen, and I say that as someone who's been working out in health clubs since 1980.

So I've given up on the notion that I can talk anyone out of doing those exercises. And I'm not even convinced they're as pointless as I once thought. Oversized arm muscles are so ingrained in physical culture that you don't really look like a lifter until your arms have the kind of thickness you can't get without curls and extensions.

So rather than fight a losing battle, I just want to put them in their place: at the end of the workout, when you've finished all the important work.

RISE OF THE MACHINES

THE ORIGINAL SIN OF BODYBUILDING

Once upon a time there was a place called Muscle Beach. Although it was a real place in Santa Monica, California, and it really was a magnet for some of the most influential fitness icons who ever walked the earth, it still seems more mythical than real. Jack LaLanne was a regular. He went on to star in the first-ever fitness show on TV, and probably introduced more people to exercise than anyone before or since. So was Steve Reeves, the first real muscleman to become a movie star. So was Joe Gold, who built the original Gold's Gym in Venice Beach; Arnold Schwarzenegger was just one of the bodybuilding champions of the '60s and '70s who trained there. So was Vic Tanny, who created the first franchised gym chain, and whose business model is still used today (for better and for worse).

Harold Zinkin was also a regular. Although you've probably never heard of him, Zinkin embodied everything that was great about Muscle Beach. He was one of the stars of the acrobatic displays that drew crowds and made the place world-famous. He was also a bodybuilding and weightlifting star. In fact, on one weekend in 1945 he won an AAU weightlifting championship on Saturday and finished second in the Mr. America bodybuilding contest on Sunday. At a time when people still thought strength training left you slow and muscle-bound, here was a guy who could lift or pose with anyone, and who also had the flexibility and balance of a world-class gymnast.

Today Zinkin is best known for inventing the Universal Gym Machine, the first multistation exercise device. I can still remember my older brother describing the wonder of a selectorized weight-stack machine, which he saw for the first time in his high school's weight room. "You change weights by moving a pin!" he told me. It sounded like something out of *Star Trek*. The weights we had at home were so crappy (we needed a wrench to use the collars on our dumbbell handles), and our progress was so slow, that we assumed a shiny machine just had to be better.

The first chance I got to use this magic machine was at my own high school in rural Missouri. A group of us who played football in the fall stayed after school during basketball and baseball seasons to work out on the machine, which occupied a former storage room adjacent to the gym. All I remember about our workouts is that I did pullups, using the bar in the doorway, to warm up for lat pulldowns. I also remember that I could do a lot of pushups back then, but again only to warm up for the *real* workout, which included chest and shoulder presses on the machine.

I held on to that fascination with machines through college. But as I graduated from campus gyms to commercial health clubs, and from storefront clubs to muscle megaplexes, I spent less time on machines and focused most of my energy on lifting barbells and dumbbells. This despite the fact that the newer, shinier gyms had more machines than I could have imagined back in high school, when I first fell in love with selectorized weights.

Over time I came to despise all but the cable machines (you'll see lots of cable exercises in Part Three) for these reasons.

Machines don't move the way your body moves. When you lift a barbell, no matter if you're pulling it off the floor or pushing it off your chest, it doesn't move straight up and down. The trajectory will be slightly different for each of us. Pressing machines typically force every lifter to push the bar along a fixed, unnatural path.

Machines don't use your muscles the way your body wants to use them. Throughout this chapter I've made an argument for using muscles in coordinated action. When you perform a full-body lift like an overhead press, squat, or deadlift, or even a basic pushup with good form, you use more muscles than anyone would ever list, including a few most of us don't know we have. Machines take most of those supporting muscles out of the movement, since the mechanism does all the balancing for you.

Machines create artificial movement patterns. Nothing you do in sports or everyday movement resembles a leg extension or leg curl. Even further afield are the movements you perform on abduction and adduction machines. (You spread your legs apart on the first, and bring your knees together on the second.) The leg press superficially resembles a jumping movement, except you'd never actually jump with your torso at a 90-degree angle to your legs. No matter how strong you get on those exercises, the strength isn't likely to translate to performance in anything you care about.

Machines put unnatural stress on your joints. A complete beginner who joins Planet Fitness and works out exclusively on machines is probably not at much risk of injury. Chances are, he'll increase his strength and muscle size and perhaps get a little leaner as well. That is, he'll get exactly what he wants from his workouts without having to worry about the learning curve that comes with using free weights. He may even gain enough confidence to learn those exercises—the equivalent of riding a bike without training wheels.

The problems arise when an ambitious lifter uses machines for serious workouts. The seated leg extension, for example, creates an unnatural strain on the knee joints. The leg press allows you to lift far more than you can on any other exercise, but with a hidden cost to your lower back: It shifts out of its natural arch as you lower an extremely heavy weight, which means you begin each repetition with your back in a weakened, vulnerable position.

I could go on, but all the examples lead back to the same basic point: When you lift a heavy weight from an unnatural position, or through an unnatural range of motion, you disable the mechanisms that would ordinarily protect your joints.

Having said all that, you probably wonder why your health club has so many expensive machines and comparatively few free weights. It's not just because it's a great marketing tool, creating the illusion of value to prospective members—although that's certainly a big factor. There are other reasons.

They're easy to use. This is a clear benefit for beginners and timid regulars. But it's also attractive to those who don't want to plan their workouts, or think about training in any analytical way. They just want to show up, do exercises in whatever order the gym has arranged the machines, and move on to the next item on the to-do list.

They allow you to focus more on individual muscles. If you're a bodybuilder, what matters most: moving like an athlete, or packing your body with muscles that ripple and bulge from every possible angle? Bodybuilders want as much stress as possible on the targeted muscles, even if it means less stress on muscles that would otherwise provide support. This is a painstaking, time-consuming approach, but yet again that's more of a feature for someone who wants to spend an hour or two a day in the weight room.

They don't require balance and coordination. When you're deep into a workout and your body is thoroughly exhausted, your coordination will be compromised. At that point, it might be safer to use a machine that provides the support your tired muscles can no longer muster.

Put another way, machine exercises aren't always a terrible choice, and free-weight exercises aren't always better than their closest machine equivalents. But that doesn't mean the two are equal. In the Lean Muscle Plan workouts, you'll start with the exercises that use the most muscle, require the most focus, develop the most useful strength, and take the most out of you. Then you'll move on to the next-best exercises, where machines will sometimes be an option.

Or to put it yet another way: You can certainly build a great physique without ever using a machine. But good luck trying to do it without ever touching free weights. The best example is probably Harold Zinkin himself. Long before he invented the multistation gym, he made himself into a champion weightlifter and bodybuilder, and a world-class acrobat, with good old-fashioned barbells, dumbbells, and body-weight exercises.

CHAPTER 4:

WHY IT'S SO FREAKIN' HARD TO GET THE BODY YOU WANT

IN A JUST AND FAIR WORLD, each of us would begin life with the same potential for strength, muscularity, body composition, and sports skill. You would choose the quality you're most interested in pursuing, and if you work the hardest and most consistently, you would achieve the best results. *You* can be the guy who hits the home run, or scores the touchdown, or ends up on the cover of a book like *The Lean Muscle Diet*.

We all know that world doesn't exist. And there's no point pretending it does. Don't get me wrong: Optimism is great to have; it's probably the number-one quality you need to launch a new training program, especially if it's your first serious attempt. I just want to make sure you have realistic expectations of what is and isn't possible, given both your individual traits and the basic limits of human physiology.

This chapter covers both. First we'll look at the power of your genes—that is, the parts of your makeup that were more or less determined the moment Daddy's swim team took gold in the Ovulation Games. The second half looks at challenges you'll encounter as a consequence of working hard to change the body your parents created. You can look at them as the price of success.

The Gene Genie

Let's start with something simple: your body mass index, or BMI. This is a ratio of weight to height. It doesn't tell us anything about your body-fat percentage, or strength, or endurance, or how charming you are at holiday parties. It's just a basic measure of how big you are relative to your height. For a male who's 5-foot-10, here are the weight ranges for each BMI category.

BMI	WEIGHT IN POUNDS	TECHNICAL CLASSIFICATION	REAL-WORLD DESCRIPTION
<18.5	<129	"Underweight"	"Somebody give that man a cheeseburger!"
18.5–24.9	129–173	"Normal weight"	The range here is enormous: from counting-ribs-skinny to lean and fit
25–29.9	174–208	"Overweight"	Anything from solid and muscular to "gettin' kinda chunky there, bro"
30–34.9	209–243	"Moderately obese"	Although most guys in this range will look fat, it includes a lot of elite athletes, including football players, bodybuilders, and powerlifters
>34.9	>243	"Severely obese"	From "wide load" to "when's the last time you counted your toes to make sure they're all still there?"

Most of you reading this want to shift your weight up or down one classification. I was born into the "normal weight" category but always considered myself skinny. It took many years in the weight room, and tons of food, to work my way up to "overweight." But even at my heaviest, and fattest, I was nowhere near "obese." Meanwhile, a lot of you came into this world predisposed to struggle with your weight. Even if you eat carefully and work out religiously, you're still the guys nobody wants to sit next to on the airplane. And you wonder, with good cause, why weight control seems so much harder for you than it is for naturally skinny bastards like me.

It's not your imagination. A study in the *International Journal of Obesity* found that more than three-fifths of your BMI is determined by your genes. The researchers came to this conclusion after looking at three types of siblings.

- Identical twins

- Nonidentical twins

- "Virtual" twins—unrelated children (one of whom is adopted) who are the same age and raised in the same family, sharing the same meals and the same environment

The exact numbers: Fully "63.6 percent of the total variance in BMI was explained by a . . . genetic component." About 25 percent was explained by environment; the rest was whatever—for example, activity levels, food preferences, and smoking. (The subjects were a mix of children and adults.)

And that's just one thing: your weight relative to your height. (Height, for what it's worth, is 80 percent genetic.) Your abilities to put on muscle, build strength, lose fat, or develop endurance are also genetically determined to some extent.

Muscle Size and Strength

Long before scientists came up with ways to look at muscle tissue at the cellular and genetic levels, muscleheads understood that some people are just born strong. Consider Paul Anderson. As a teenager in the 1940s, he wanted to get stronger for football. With no coaching beyond some magazines and an enthusiastic brother-in-law, he put together his own backyard workouts with equipment he scavenged from junkyards. Those workouts made him strong enough to earn a football scholarship to Furman University. There, in his first encounter with a real barbell, Anderson knocked out a set of 10 squats with 350 pounds. Thus began a strength career that included the 1956 Olympic gold medal in weightlifting (he was the last American to win as a super heavyweight) and countless feats of superhuman strength.

Anderson isn't the only one. Gym lore gives us lots of stories about powerlifting and bodybuilding champions who began with extraordinary strength, or who gained dozens of pounds of lean muscle before they injected their first steroids. Where does natural strength like that come from, assuming Planet Krypton is fictional?

The bones, for starters. A pound of bone can support a maximum of 5 pounds of muscle, so big-boned boys have a decisive advantage. (You can add some bone mass with a good strength program, which I'll explain in more detail in Part Three.)

Proportions also matter. Strength, for example, is about leverage. The best bench pressers will have relatively short arms and thick chests. Those features shorten the distance the bar has to travel. For the same reason, the strongest squatter will have short, thick legs. And the best deadlifter will have relatively long arms; since his hands start closer to the floor, he doesn't have to pull the bar as far to complete the lift.

For muscular aesthetics, the key is the length of your muscles—where the muscle belly ends and the tendon begins. The easiest example is the biceps.

Flex your left biceps so your forearm and upper arm are at a 90-degree angle. Now use the fingers of your right hand to measure the distance between the end of the biceps and your forearm. If you can fit just one finger into that space, you're in luck. You've hit the short-tendon lottery. That means your biceps, when fully developed, will be long and thick. I, on the other hand, can fit two fingers into that space on my own arm, with room to spread them out. The gap is almost wide enough for three fingers. Combine that with relatively long arms, and I'm left with exactly zero chance for a successful career in competitive bodybuilding. If I didn't know how to type, I'd have no career options at all!

The same holds true for every other muscle you care about. You can make it bigger with training, but what it looks like when it's fully developed depends on structural factors that are out of your control. This is especially disappointing for those who struggle to get as lean as humanly possible, only to discover their newly revealed abs have an odd appearance.

But what does "fully developed" even mean? Is it determined by how much work you're willing to put in? Once again, I'm sorry to say, it's not that fair or straightforward. Let's say you recruit a few dozen people who swear on a stack of Bibles that they haven't lifted weights in the past 5 years. And let's say you give all those people an identical training program and monitor them closely for 16 weeks to make sure everyone appears to put in about the same effort.

A research team at the University of Alabama-Birmingham did exactly that and found that the study's subjects fit into three distinct categories. On the "woo-hoo!" end of the spectrum were the extreme responders. The fibers in their thigh muscles got 50 percent bigger. On the "of all the Charlie Browns in the world, you're the Charlie Browniest" end were those whose muscles didn't grow at all. In between was a Goldilocks group whose thigh-muscle fibers grew by 25 percent.

Here's the interesting part: The results were predictable. Who gains the most mass is largely determined by who starts with the most satellite cells, which provide supplemental nuclei to muscle fibers for growth and repairs. Some people have a lot. Most of us have moderate amounts. And some poor bastards have comparatively few.

None of the subjects, we assume, had an inkling of their superior muscle-building potential. If they did, you have to think they would have been training all along. Who wouldn't want more muscle, especially when you know the results are virtually guaranteed, thanks to a winning genetic predisposition? It's like Calvinism for meatheads.

Stamina, Endurance, and Athleticism

I once had a really awkward conversation with an author whose workout book I was editing. He was a former pro athlete who segued into modeling. It's hard to describe how impossibly lean, muscular, and good-looking this guy was without coming off like I'm plagiarizing a romance novel. Like his father, he was immediately elite at every sport he played. But he also had challenges that made his story interesting. His father had died young from a heart attack. Most of his siblings were obese, and some had major health problems. His own athletic prowess was handicapped by congenital back and knee problems, on top of a self-destructive streak that he'd worked hard to overcome.

So his story was inspiring, his physique was amazing, and his workout program was solid. The awkward conversation grew out of something else: his insistence that any reader could achieve the same results if he just wanted it enough. I explained to him that the average person doesn't have a fraction of his physique-building potential. Hardly anyone can put on that much mass without also adding a lot of fat. And even fewer people can get cover-model lean without sacrificing whatever muscle they began with.

He protested that he worked hard to get in camera-ready shape. I agreed, and his work ethic was indeed admirable. His typical routine was an hour-long strength workout followed by an hour of full-court basketball, sprint intervals, or something equally grueling. But yet again, his ability to work out for hours a day, every day, isn't shared by the genetically inferior. I told him I'd love to be able to work out that hard and that often, but it would kill me. My max for serious lifting is three good workouts a week, and I needed at least a full day to recover from an hour of pickup basketball.

To say I caught him by surprise is an understatement. In all his years of being the strongest, fastest, leanest, and best-looking guy in the room, no matter which room he happened to be in, it never crossed his mind that his ability to train hard almost every day of his life was unique. He just thought he was more dedicated than everyone else.

Research backs me up. Look at any population, and you'll find a vast range of abilities. But within that mix you'll find two specific types of outliers. Some start out with a high level of endurance. Without any training, they could go out and run circles around most of us. And some respond to training more favorably. That is, on day one of the program we might all be equally bad at an endurance challenge. But after a few workouts these super responders will leave us in the dust.

The athlete-model had some crazy combination of those traits. First, he was instantly better at just about anything he tried. Second, he improved faster than the average mortal, in part because he had the stamina to practice more, and practice longer, and still recover well enough to do it again the next day, and the day after. Add to that his otherworldly ability to pack on muscle while staying super lean, and you have a guy who's a genetic freak on multiple levels. Even with all that going for him, he wouldn't have been successful as a model if not for his facial symmetry and bone structure. And I haven't even mentioned the fact that he was several inches taller than average.

A guy like that can inspire people to grind through adversity, and he can certainly offer great workout advice. Just because he has great genetics doesn't mean he hasn't learned a lot of important lessons about how to train for specific results. My point to him was that he couldn't teach anybody how to be just like him when it's almost a miracle that someone like him exists at all.

Body Fat

All these things are regulated, in part, by your genes:

▶ How much fat you have

▶ Where you have it

- How much food you want to eat

- How your body uses that food

- How much of that food your body burns during digestion

- How much exercise you do habitually

- How many calories your body burns during that exercise

In my many years of writing about exercise, nutrition, and weight control, I typically see a bipolar reaction to information like this. Most people cry foul, saying that genetics is a lousy excuse for being fat and sedentary, or skinny and weak, or whatever the problem is. Many of them, especially my friends in the fitness industry, believe their own results are proof that anyone can overcome the lousy hand he was dealt *if he just sacks up and gets the work done.* Just about all of them believe their own genetics were either irrelevant or a handicap to be mastered by brute willpower. So it follows that their magnificent physiques and athletic accomplishments are proof of their testicular density, as well as a rebuke to all those who are too lazy to achieve the same results.

But the truth is more nuanced. No one in pro sports or at the elite levels of bodybuilding or powerlifting started out with inferior genes for the traits they depend on for a living. Of course they worked hard, and that's impressive. They also may have had terrible difficulties in other areas. I'll give you an extreme example. You would think that in a sport like pro basketball, height and athleticism trump all other variables. But even among tall, athletic men, other factors come into play. More NBA players come from affluent neighborhoods and fewer are born out of wedlock or to young mothers than you'd expect. In other words, the factors that give you an edge in any line of work—a stable family with resources to invest in your development—also matter in pro sports. We can never assume that someone with great genetics had an easy path to success. But we also can't pretend his great genetics didn't matter.

A few people, including me, take the opposite position. With each new study we gain a deeper appreciation of the challenges some individuals face when they try to change their bodies with diet and exercise. Acknowledging those difficulties makes their eventual success even more exciting.

No one thinks genetics account for 100 percent of a person's weight or body composition. I don't think I've ever met a healthy person who was incapable of getting leaner and stronger. The fact you're hungrier than the average person isn't an excuse to eat loads of crap. Alan and I wouldn't have written *The Lean Muscle Diet* if we didn't think our readers could make major and sometimes even remarkable transformations. But we all have to be realistic about the limitations our bodies impose. There's no point pressuring yourself to achieve a shape that isn't in the cards for you.

The Price of Success

Every serious lifter remembers the first time everything clicks. Strength improves from one workout to the next. Muscles grow so fast, friends ask if you've been spending time at the local antiaging clinic. Fat melts. In the fitness biz we call them "newbie gains," but they can also happen to experienced lifters who try a new diet or a different style of training.

I'll offer a shamelessly self-serving example. Let's say you've been working out the past few years with a program of your own design. It started with bits and pieces from the program a trainer gave you when you joined the gym, which you modified based on an article you once read on bodybuilding.com, and then augmented with random exercises you see the gym's biggest guys doing. Then one day you pick up a book called *The Lean Muscle Diet* and start over with the workouts you see in Part Three. Overnight, it seems, you've found your way back onto Hypertrophy Highway, with impressive strength gains and a shrinking waistline thanks to Alan's diet plan.

You cruise for a while, thinking you've finally cracked the code. You'll never struggle again! But around the 6-month mark, you notice the gains aren't coming as fast anymore. And by the end of the year, you realize you've actually regained a little of the fat you lost. What you once thought would be the perfect plan for the rest of your life turns out to have an expiration date.

On the other hand, if you're a bona fide newb, and this is your first training program, your steady improvements will probably continue for a year or two. The fastest gains might not even come right at the beginning; there's a learning curve to the exercises, as I'll explain in more detail in the workout chapters. There's also a series of neural adaptations your body makes before the hypertrophy mechanisms fully engage. That's one of the reasons why your strength improves so much faster than your muscle size early in a program. (That, and the fact that any strength gains are measurable, while hypertrophy tends to be more a matter of perception and guesswork: A true beginner might simultaneously lose fat and gain muscle, which means his body is shrinking despite the fact his muscles are growing.)

I can't guess when any individual will hit the sweet spot, how big the gains will be, or how long they will continue. All I can promise is that they will eventually slow down. Each of us has a genetic ceiling. We just don't know where it is until we reach it. But even then, the gains don't stop entirely until you quit trying. The extreme example is elite Olympic weightlifters. Studies back in the '80s showed that their improvements were tiny: just 1.5 to 2 percent a year in their lifts, and 1 percent in lean muscle mass. At the same time they lost about 1 to 2 percent of their fat per year. For you or me, that would be a terrible return for a year's worth of training. But for one of them, it might be enough to get on the podium for the first time.

Your results may come quickly or slowly. (We'll show you the range you can expect in Chapter 5.) You may lose 5 pounds your first week on Alan's diet, which would be terrific. Or you may wonder why you can't lose even 1 a week. If this chapter serves any purpose at all, it's to convince you not to compare your results to anyone else's. A lot of the guys reading this will fall under the dreaded skinny-fat rubric, with a relatively small frame, low muscle mass, and a high percentage of fat. The only way to transform yourself from both skinny and fat to neither skinny nor fat is with a long, erratic, and sometimes frustrating process. Muscle is your body's best tool for chipping away at fat. But you can't use what you don't yet have.

I say this with full conviction, and you won't find an expert to contradict me: You're going to have to build your new body from the inside out, starting with the structural exercises that develop strong bones and connective tissues as well as strong, versatile muscles. I'll explain it in more detail in Chapter 9, but for now, please take my word that this process can't be rushed.

Conversely, some of you will have a lot of fat to lose, but with a lot of muscle beneath it and a strong frame to support the muscle. Progress may come quickly, enabled by the fact that your XXL body uses more energy than someone smaller will burn doing the exact same things.

In fact, you may lose weight so fast that you run smack into one of the most vexing problems of all.

When Your Body Thinks It's Too Stupid to Eat

People who go on a fast for the first time expect to feel terrible. Instead, many report that they feel more awake and alert. It's like they've found a new gear they didn't know they had. This makes perfect sense in an evolutionary context.

Imagine a Stone Age man who's starving. He hasn't been able to feed his family for days. Will his body shut down to conserve energy? Or will it give him an extra jolt of adrenaline to help him find something to eat?

Now suppose the same man is struggling through a rough year. A year ago there was plenty to hunt and gather. Now, thanks to a drought, there are fewer plants, and the ones that survive yield less. As the vegetation withers, the herbivores move on. These include the big, meaty animals like horses, bison, and deer. The small game is still around, but those animals are smaller and faster, and thus harder to hunt and kill. Worse, it takes dozens of them to provide the nutrition of a single antelope. Then there's the competition from both land and air. Those wolves and eagles are superpredators with distinct advantages over humans, who mostly evolved to gather and scavenge. And to make it even worse, the bigger carnivores—bears, lions, and saber-toothed cats—are still around. They not only compete with cavemen for the remaining food, they also aren't averse to snacking on the occasional manwich until something more substantial comes along.

The caveman's body is no longer cranking out stress hormones to help him through a temporary crisis. That would be a terrible use of his diminished energy supply. Instead, his metabolism downshifts. Now he needs fewer calories to get through a typical day, and when he has to move more than usual—on a multiday hunt, for example—his muscles burn less energy per mile. This is over and above the fact that his depleted body is lighter than it was before, and thus uses fewer calories anyway.

This metabolic slowdown is called *adaptive thermogenesis.* As a survival mechanism it makes sense to use less energy when you have less food to eat. But you aren't a caveman, and your weight loss has nothing to do with survival, unless the goal is to live longer by weighing less.

This is what happens.

> **1.** A body that weighs less will burn fewer calories at rest, as you'd expect. But the math gets skewed when you lose

weight. The decline in your resting metabolism is steeper than it should be, based on the number of pounds you've lost.

2. A weight-reduced body will also burn fewer calories during exercise. So even though your training goal is to burn calories you've already stored, your body reacts as if you're searching for *more* calories, with no idea when or where you'll find them.

3. The less you eat, the hungrier you get. Hunger hormones like ghrelin upregulate, while satiety hormones like leptin—the ones that give you that nice "all full" feeling following a meal—have less potency. You want to eat not only more, but also more often.

4. While these mechanisms make sense for the survival of a species that often had to deal with prolonged scarcity, they're brutal when food is rarely more than a few feet away. But, to paraphrase a former high-ranking official, you go to weight loss with the body you have, not the body you might want or wish to have at a later time.

All this works in reverse when you're trying to gain weight. The new muscle tissue is more metabolically active than fat tissue when you put it to use in your workouts. The more muscle you have, the more energy your body uses during and after workouts. The more you eat, the more your body burns during digestion. And some of us are genetically predisposed to move more—to fidget, basically—when we eat more, and thus have excess energy floating around. So even though we're trying as hard as we can to gain weight, our bodies are fighting back.

The two processes, while parallel, don't seem to work with equal potency. A body that's resistant to weight gain won't work quite as hard to maintain homeostasis as a body that's trying to resist weight loss. But the principle is the same, and it's a recurring theme throughout *The Lean Muscle Diet*: Your body does what it can to keep what it has. You have to work that much harder to make your body change, and to make sure it stays changed.

That's why Alan and I base our plan on eating, training, and acting *as if you already have* the body you want to have. You can't change your genes, but you can change the food and activities that your genes act upon.

How to Be Smarter Than Your Metabolism

The fact your body fights back against weight change isn't a surprise. It's a survival mechanism, and for most of human history it did its job pretty well. Consider how your body generates energy when you cut off all or most of your food.

1. First it uses the most easily accessible energy, which is the fat and carbohydrate you have in your blood, your muscles, and your liver.

2. Your body's carbohydrate stores will run down quickly if you don't replenish them, and your body can't function without some in your system. So the longer you go without eating, the more your body will shift toward using stored fat for energy, a process called *lipolysis*. The supply you keep in your fat cells, even if you're relatively lean, is enough to keep you going for months.

3. But your body will also protect against losing too much fat, since it needs a baseline amount to keep you alive. When that baseline is threatened, your body will shift to using the protein stored in your muscles, converting it to energy through a process called *proteolysis*. The equivalent would be a pioneer family caught inside during a snowstorm. As they run out of fuel to keep their hearth going, they resort to chopping up and burning their furniture.

4. Burning the muscles—or the furniture—isn't the last resort. That comes when your body starts using structural proteins, like those in your skin, organs, bones, or connective tissues.

Of course, your metabolism is going to slow down dramatically the further you go in this process. If you were actually starving, it would want to delay the inevitable as long as possible. This is why rapid weight loss—usually defined as more than 2 pounds a week—is rarely advisable for anyone who isn't severely obese. And it's rarely sustainable for anyone beyond the first few weeks. When your metabolism doesn't have time to adjust to the new, lower weight, it will do everything it can to return to the weight it considers normal.

To keep your metabolism from slowing down too far, your first and most important tool is protein. Because it takes more energy to digest, it keeps your metabolism elevated. It also supports lean tissue. It's inevitable that you will lose some muscle when you shed a lot of weight, but protein helps you keep as much as possible.

The other tool: vigorous exercise. To quote from a paper on adaptive thermogenesis by two of its preeminent researchers, Michael Rosenbaum and Rudolph Leibel, both of Columbia University: "[M]aintenance of a reduced body weight is associated with an approximate 20 percent increase in skeletal muscle work efficiency *at low levels of exercise.*" (Emphasis mine.)

In this context, remember that efficiency is bad; you want your muscles to be inefficient, to use *more* energy. Moving along at a slow, steady pace lends itself to increased efficiency. It's the equivalent of retooling a car engine to get more miles per gallon.

I don't want to imply that shorter, higher-intensity exercise bouts are necessarily better than slower, continuous workouts for weight loss. The evidence doesn't really support that. You can burn calories with either type of exercise. Any of us will burn the most with the exercise we like the most, which is the one we're most likely to stick with for long enough to see results.

But if you've already lost some weight and your body is predisposed to burning fewer calories with steady-pace exercise, then an obvious play is to find ways to make the exercise less predictable. There's nothing more inefficient than running fast or lifting heavy objects in relatively short bursts of effort, broken up by rest periods of varying lengths.

Keep in mind that if you're counting on exercise as your sole or primary weight loss tool, you've given yourself a pretty steep challenge no matter how you attempt it. Controlling what you eat, and how much, will have a much larger effect for most of us.

That's exactly what we'll tackle in Part Two.

FACT-CHECKING CONVENTIONAL WISDOM

MY, WHAT BIG CLICHÉS YOU HAVE

Like every other subculture, the fitness world has a stockpile of clichés for every situation. Some are motivational. Some are prescriptive. Some are repeated because they make perfect sense. Others only sound good because the people who repeat them look good and seem to know what they're talking about. Let's start with the one that bothers me more than any other.

"Abs are made in the kitchen."

I started hearing this one about the time that fitness advocates came to grips with an inconvenient truth: Exercise by itself, with no change in diet, simply isn't very effective for weight loss. Almost overnight, as I recall, trainers went from scolding people about not training hard enough to scolding them about not dieting hard enough. Shortly after this I noticed the rise of what I call stunt dieting among fitness pros. Being on a disciplined, restrictive diet was no longer enough—it had to be a raw-food diet, with extended periods of fasting, and no wiggle room unless it's a planned cheat day, in which case the trainer makes a calculated decision to eat a dozen hot-fudge sundaes soaked in bacon fat. And then shares the experience on Instagram.

It has multiple corollaries, including "You can't out-train a bad diet" and "Diet is 90 percent of the battle."

Here's my counterargument.

Take a pair of identical twins. Give one of them a perfect diet but no exercise. Give the other a fantastic workout program but let him eat whatever he wants. Which one will have a better physique in 12 months? I think it would depend on their genes. If they tend to be lean without much effort, then the training twin will probably look a lot better. If they are genetically on the thick side, I'd put my money on the one who diets.

But in pretending it's one or the other, I'm making the same mistake as the guys I disagree with. A strong, athletic, muscular body can only be the result of hard training and smart eating. That's why I like this version of the quote from bodybuilding legend Dave Draper: "What you eat is what you get." Eat a lean and healthy diet to get a lean and healthy body. Eat crap . . . well, you get the idea.

"Pain is weakness leaving the body."

If you're an elite, competitive athlete, you really do have to play hurt and occasionally push yourself to the absolute limits of human perseverance. You're making a calculated risk that winning now is more important than the price you'll pay down the road.

But for the rest of us, I like this rebuttal by my friend Rannoch Donald on Facebook: "Pain is not weakness leaving the body. It's a protective mechanism that, when ignored, will simply turn up the volume until you have to pay attention. Good luck with that."

The more popular version of that quote—"No pain, no gain"—is only slightly less insidious. It's perfectly reasonable if you modify it to say, "You won't get the results you want if you never push yourself outside your comfort zone." I think every athlete and fitness enthusiast would agree. But to some people, "discomfort" and "pain" are synonyms, so it's possible that, for them, "no pain, no gain" is mostly accurate.

"Winners never quit, and quitters never win."

"Winners quit all the time," writes Seth Godin in *The Dip: A Little Book That Teaches You When to Quit (and When to Stick)*. "They just quit the right stuff at the right time." That quote is on the book's first page. The rest of the book is about how to know when to stick it out through rough times (the titular dip) and when to cut your losses and move on to the next opportunity. The difference between life's winners and losers, he argues, is that the most successful quit fast and quit decisively when they realize they've hit a dead end. The least successful either stay in that no-win situation, or they give up too soon, mistaking a dip for a dead end.

As someone who's quit (or been fired from) a long list of jobs that weren't right for me, along with quite a few sports and fitness activities that didn't click, I was attracted to Godin's premise. What I didn't expect to find was this comment on the one form of exercise I've stuck with for most of my life:

"Weight training is a fascinating science. Basically, you do a minute or two of work . . . so that the last few seconds of work will cause that muscle to grow." Those who don't get the benefits of lifting, he observes, might put in the same time as the ones who succeed. But they fail to push themselves during those sets and reps that make all the difference.

"You just have to want it."

This is a corollary to the "winners never quit" fallacy. While not quite as dumb as "you have to give 110 percent" (which is motivating only if you're bad at math), it's still just partially true. It's not enough to want something. What you want is meaningless. Wanting it doesn't mean you have any chance at success, that it's right for you, or that it's right for the people in your life. You may know somebody who chose the pursuit of a sport or fitness goal over his family.

In my experience, success occurs when what you *want* intersects with what you *need.* How do you know what you need? You just do. Eventually.

Now here are three clichés I happen to like a lot.

"Lift weights, not ego."

This is a variation on "leave your ego at the door," which I've never liked much. Freud notwithstanding, most of us equate ego with vanity, and vanity with pride. I happen to think pride is highly underrated, at least compared with the other deadly sins (especially greed, sloth, and gluttony). Pride gets us into the weight room in the first place, and pride is what keeps us rolling with a disciplined diet and training program.

However, once you're *in* the gym, you have to remember why you're there: to train, not to preen. There's a difference between developing strength and demonstrating it. Focus on what you're trying to accomplish, rather than demonstrating what you've already achieved.

"Don't fit yourself to the exercise. Fit the exercise to you."

I don't think this admonition, which I saw in an article about deadlifts by Nick Tumminello, has reached the gym-rat demographic. So it's probably not yet a cliché. But it's damned good advice. I've made the mistake of including exercises in my workouts that hurt to perform, or that clearly weren't a good fit for my body or my abilities at that time. I used to do this in my workout books as well, but stopped when I realized most of my questions from readers asked if they could substitute another exercise for one that made their joints angry or their orthopedists happy. That's why almost every exercise you'll find in Part Three has optional modifications or alternatives. The goal is to use basic movement patterns to develop muscular size and strength, not to master specific exercises.

"The best workout for you is the one you haven't tried."
Here's my all-time favorite bit of weight-room wisdom, and the reason I write books: to help lifters find a system that's better than the one they're currently using. It of course assumes that what you're doing now *isn't* working for you, but that's not the only reason to switch up your program. That's why I also like this alt version: "If you do what you've always done, you get what you already have." A lot of you are looking for something that builds on what you already have. And now you've found it.

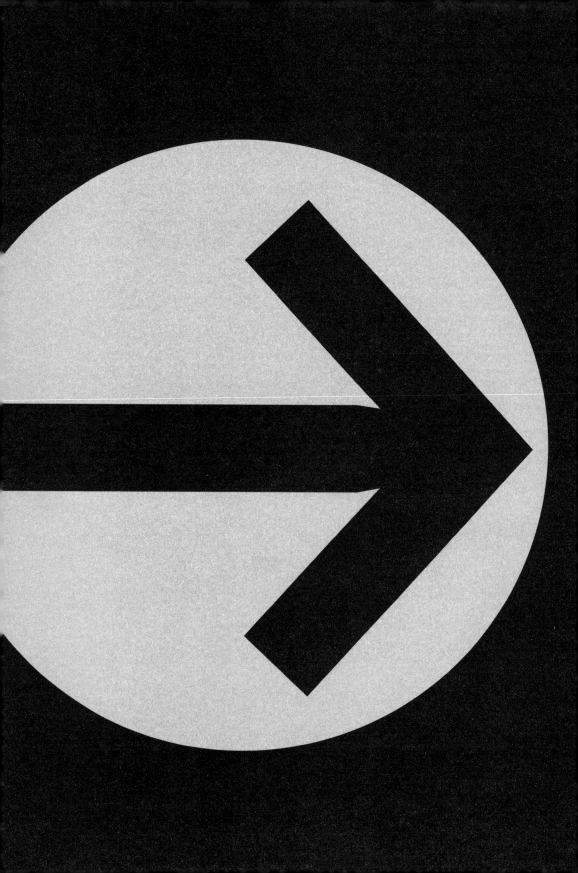

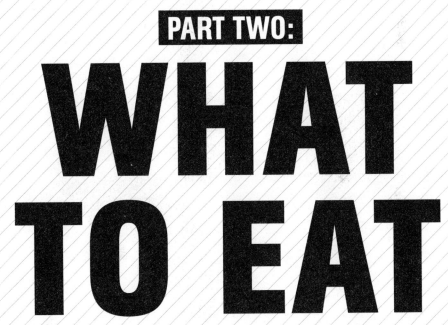

PART TWO:

WHAT TO EAT

CHAPTER 5

THE ONE WITH ALL THE MATH

YOU'VE HEARD THE CLICHÉS: "A journey of a thousand miles begins with a single step." "The journey is the reward." "Happiness is a journey, not a destination." They're clichés for a reason: They sound good, but they don't actually help you accomplish anything specific. Which brings to mind a great Yogi Berra quote: "If you don't know where you're going, you'll end up someplace else."

The key to Alan's diet plan is to know exactly where you're going—that is, to start with a target body weight (TBW), which by definition must be a specific number. Even if you have a TBW in mind, please read the following sections carefully to see if that target is realistic. Our assumption is that you're committed to a 6-month training and diet program.

The Fat Loss Continuum

Alan uses four broad categories of weight loss goals.

A. Rapid weight gain with potentially significant fat gain

B. Muscle gain with minimal fat gain

C. Fat loss with minimal muscle loss

D. Rapid weight loss with potentially significant muscle loss

Since a journey of 26 letters begins with A, let's start there. Rapid weight gain is rarely the subject of high-level research. With only a handful of exceptions, that territory was long ago conceded to high school football coaches, bodybuilding gurus, and self-taught endocrinologists, aka steroid enthusiasts. We assume some overlap in those three groups.

In one classic study, James Levine and colleagues at the Mayo Clinic deliberately overfed nonobese men by 1,000 calories a day for 8 weeks, the equivalent of adding four McDonald's hamburgers every day without changing anything else. Since a pound of fat contains 3,500 calories of stored energy, basic math tells you that adding 7,000 calories a week, with no additional exercise, should produce 2 pounds of fat. Over 8 weeks that's 16 pounds.

That's not what happened. Lots of calories were burned off through a previously unnamed process Dr. Levine called *nonexercise-activity thermogenesis,* or NEAT. NEAT can be any type of movement, conscious or unconscious, including thrashing around in your sleep. Because of NEAT, volunteers gained an average of just 10 pounds.

And that's still only half the story. The NEAT range was enormous. One volunteer burned 692 more calories while overeating. He turned into a hummingbird; his body did everything short of spontaneous liposuction to maintain his original weight. If you believe you're resistant to weight gain (in the bodybuilding world, the term of art is "hardgainer"), it's probably not your imagination. There's a good chance you're a NEAT freak.

Another volunteer burned 98 *fewer* calories. His body actually slowed down, as if to make it easier for the calories to find a comfortable resting place. Guys like him often end up at point D on the continuum: seeking rapid weight loss, even if it means losing some muscle along with fat.

That trade-off isn't as bad as you think. Even when obese people are given just 400 to 800 calories a day—a typical lunch for most of us—they lose 75 percent fat and 25 percent lean mass. The more fat they have, the more they lose. Even better, the more weight they lose initially and the faster they lose it, the better their success in keeping it off.

Common sense would tell you that someone who's already lean would lose a higher percentage of muscle during rapid weight loss. Indeed, that's what a Norwegian team found when they tested fast versus slow weight loss in elite athletes. The ones who lost 1.4 percent of their weight per week sacrificed more lean mass than the ones who reduced at half that rate. Amazingly, some of the subjects actually *gained* muscle during the slow weight loss, which for most people is the physiological equivalent of winning the lottery. It happens under two conditions.

▶ The person is both overweight and new to strength training

▶ The person tries a new program that offers a novel muscle-building stimulus

In the Norwegian study, the muscle gainers were endurance athletes who weren't used to strength training. So any lifting program would have been a novel stimulus. Most of you, we suspect, will be after one of the two goals in the middle: B (muscle gain with minimal fat gain) or C (fat loss with minimal muscle loss). So let's look at what you can expect.

Rate Shock

In Alan's experience, these are average results during a program that lasts 6 to 12 months.

Fat Loss with Minimal Muscle Loss

▶ 2 pounds per week in the obese (BMI of 30 or above, as explained in Chapter 4)

▶ 1 pound per week in the overweight (BMI of 25 to 30)

▶ ½ pound per week, or less, in guys who are lean and trying to get even leaner

Muscle Gain with Minimal Fat Gain

▶ 2 to 3 pounds per month in novices and advanced beginners (those with less than 2 years of consistent strength training)

▶ 1 to 2 pounds per month in intermediates (those with 2 to 4 years of consistent training)

▶ ½ pound per month in advanced lifters who are close to their genetic ceiling

The first few weeks and months will bring the biggest losses or gains, which is great for motivation. Unfortunately, early success often raises expectations, which can lead to disappointment down the road when the rate of change inevitably slows. That's why Alan likes to start with a specific TBW, and a specific amount of time to achieve it.

For contrast, consider the conventional approaches. A fictional character named Dan, who weighs 240 pounds, decides it's time for a change. Dan buys a best-selling diet book (that is, one *not* written by me) and resolves to follow the book's sample diet to the letter. He doesn't know that the sample diet is just 1,300 calories a day, or that it's less than half what he typically eats. Nor does he have a TBW in mind. He just wants to lose weight—the faster, the better.

The pounds seem to fly off Dan's body at first—24 pounds in just 6 weeks. His wife jokes that he loses a pound every time he takes a shower. In another month Dan figures he'll be under 200 pounds for the first time since his freshman year in college. But of course he never gets there. The phenomena I described in Chapter 4 have already kicked in; he just doesn't know it yet. Because he's hungry all the time, his adherence gets a little worse every day. And because he's been over 200 pounds his entire adult life, Dan's metabolism fights back. His NEAT has already declined, and with the loss of lean tissue, his resting metabolism has also downshifted.

By the time Dan finally concedes that he's no longer following the diet, he's regained some of the weight, and his body is primed to regain the rest, plus a few extra pounds. That's what happens when you toss a firecracker into the hornet's nest of homeostasis.

But suppose Dan had started with a TBW of 216 pounds, an ambitious but realistic loss of 24 pounds, or 10 percent of his starting weight. Suppose he had given himself 6 months to achieve it, rather than getting there by accident after just 6 weeks. And suppose he started with a diet plan *precisely calculated to maintain that target weight* once he achieved it. The weight loss wouldn't be linear; Dan would probably start off losing several pounds a week, and less than a pound a week at the end. But once he reached 216 pounds, there's a great chance he'd stay there. His metabolism would adjust to the TBW as he approaches it.

Would Dan be happy at 216 pounds? We hope so. A 10 percent drop is a very big deal. Weight loss in the 2 to 5 percent range has been shown to help lower blood pressure, blood sugar, and triglycerides, all of which are components of the metabolic syndrome. And there's nothing that prevents him from losing more weight down the road.

We'll say more about Dan later in the chapter, when we show you how he can reach his goals using the Lean Muscle Plan. For now, let's talk about you.

Alan's system works best when you choose a specific body-fat percentage as your goal, and then calculate how much you would weigh when you reach it. Makes sense, right? After all, if you're pursuing goal B or C—keeping your muscle while losing weight, or keeping fat in check while gaining muscle— then your target weight depends on your target body composition.

To choose a reasonable body-fat goal, you have to make two estimations: how much fat you have now, and how lean you can reasonably expect to become in 6 months. This is a part of the process you want to get right, because your success depends on it.

The Big-Ass Problem of Estimating Body Fat

The healthiest body-fat range for men is roughly 11 to 22 percent. (For women it's 20 to 33 percent.) At the lower end, just about any guy would look fit and feel good about himself. He'd also be in good company. Here are some of the body-fat percentages of elite college athletes, compiled for a classic 1983 study.

SPORT	BODY-FAT PERCENTAGE
Average college male	15
Canoe and kayak	13
Swimming	12.4
Weight-class athletes (boxing and wrestling)	6.9–7.9
Sprinting (100 and 200 meters)	6.5
Marathon	6.4

The same study today would probably find higher levels for the average student and lower levels for some of the athletes. But the trends would otherwise hold. Athletes whose weight is supported by water don't need to be as lean as sprinters, whose success depends on having maximum power-generating muscle with minimal fat, which would act as an anchor. The endurance athletes, conversely, have to sacrifice both muscle and fat in order to carry as little weight as humanly possible.

Other, more recent studies have looked at competitive bodybuilders, finding they reach 5 percent body fat by the time they hit the stage. One study followed a drug-free pro through a yearlong cycle of training and recovery. He went from 14.5 to 4.5 percent fat in 6 months. That's right: He lost more than two-thirds of his body fat in 25 weeks. And this is a guy who probably looked a lot better than you or me before he started his contest prep.

Note that today's bodybuilders are leaner than even weight-restricted boxers and wrestlers were a generation ago. That's why they look like human anatomy charts when they're in contest condition. Fitness-magazine cover models are nearly as lean, although not typically as muscular as the bodybuilders.

Five percent body fat is unachievable for most of us. But you can still look pretty good in the low double digits. You can probably achieve at least a "blurry" six-pack. In the most flattering light it might even look like the real thing.

To get to that solid, unambiguous, *hard* six-pack, the kind you see on elite athletes, you need to get down to the 7 to 9 percent range. Most young, fit guys, in Alan's experience, can get down there for a few weeks at a time. But only the genetically or pharmacologically gifted (or those whose job or sport forces them to work hard for hours a day) can hope to stay at that level year-round. And although it's below what large studies say is a healthy range, there's nothing inherently *unhealthy* about it, as long as you achieve and maintain it with serious exercise and a good diet. You could say the same about a body-fat percentage north of 22 percent. If you're training hard and eating well but are genetically predisposed to carry a wider-than-average load, you're almost certainly healthier than a sedentary junk-food eater with less body fat.

But how do you know what yours is *now*? Alan says the only truly accurate way to measure body-fat percentage is dissection. Of course we all want to look cut, but that's going a bit too far. High-tech methods include DXA and the Bod-Pod, which are used in university-level research and rarely available to the public. The easiest low-tech method is to have a trainer take skin-fold measurements with calipers. The number you get largely depends on the skill of the trainer. As for bathroom scales that purport to measure body fat via bioelectrical impedance, you're lucky if they measure your *weight* accurately. Body-fat readings are all over the place.

The simplest solution is to use an online calculator that includes measurements of your waist, hips, forearm, and wrist. Do this first thing in the morning, right after weighing yourself, and you'll get a ballpark figure that's good enough for our purposes.

Once you have a number, this is how Alan wants you to use it.

How to Choose a Target Body Weight

STEP 1: Calculate lean body mass (LBM).

Let's say you weigh 200 pounds and estimate 25 percent body fat. That means you have 50 pounds of fat and 150 pounds of lean mass.

STEP 2: Select your target LBM and multiply by 100.

Even if you have some fat to lose, you probably want to increase your lean mass. As noted earlier, a realistic target for an intermediate-level lifter is a pound a month, which would be 6 pounds in 6 months. That gives you a target LBM of 156 pounds. The next part is easy: 156 × 100 = 15,600.

STEP 3: Choose a target body-fat percentage and subtract from 100.

In Alan's experience, the following are realistic rates at which an intermediate lifter can decrease his body-fat percentage.

CURRENT STATUS	MONTHLY DECREASE IN BODY-FAT PERCENTAGE
Obese (>25% body fat)	3–4%
Overweight (20–25% body fat)	2–3%
Average (13–19% body fat)	1–2%
Lean (<13% body fat)	≤1%

At 25 percent fat, a realistic rate of decline is 2 to 3 percentage points per month, which means you could drop 13 points in 6 months, leaving you with 12 percent body fat. So, 100 − 12 = 88.

STEP 4:	Divide the result of Step 2 by the result of Step 3 to get your target body weight.

In this case, 15,600 ÷ 88 = 177.3.

This is your TBW for the 6-month diet and training program. The net loss is 22.7 pounds. But since your target weight includes 6 additional pounds of lean mass, the actual fat loss is 28.7 pounds, in about 25 weeks.

That number may look large or small to you. To Alan it looks entirely realistic. You're trying to gain a pound of muscle per month with a net weight loss of less than a pound a week. Even your most ambitious goal—shaving more than half your body's fat—is at the low end of the achievable range.

How to Calculate Daily Calories

You can find any number of ways to estimate the amount of food you need to maintain your current weight. Weight loss advice often suggests you start with that number and then deduct 500 calories a day. That's 3,500 calories a week, equal to the energy in a pound of fat. It should work at first, but it has a big flaw: It assumes weight loss is linear, which it isn't, as we explain throughout *The Lean Muscle Diet*. The standard advice also fails to take into account your TBW (assuming you have one) and your workout program. Higher-intensity training has an effect on body composition that's different from lower-intensity exercise, and body composition in turn affects your metabolism.

Alan's formula accounts for all those factors. As he sees it, your TBW is a surrogate measure for your lean mass, plus a small buffer.

The Standard Formula:
TBW x (9 – 11 + average weekly hours of training)

This formula works best for guys who are sedentary when they aren't training. It assumes a low level of NEAT. Here's how you use it.

STEP 1:	Estimate your total weekly hours of training.

Include both strength training and cardio. You can also add in recreational sports, like a challenging hike or pickup basketball game, or even physical labor if you regularly spend time landscaping or roofing. Let's say you put in 3 hours a week in the weight room, do 30 minutes of cardio twice a week, and typically play basketball for an hour on the weekend. You're otherwise sedentary when you work, commute, and catch up on *Dr. Who* episodes at home. For you, that's a total of 5 weekly hours of training.

STEP 2: Estimate your average weekly training intensity, and add this number to your average weekly training hours.

Here Alan is talking about *intensity of effort.* (The textbook definition refers to *intensity of load,* meaning the percentage of your 1-rep maximum on any given lift.) It's subjective, but high-effort training does leave traces. If you're still breathing hard for a while after you finish your workout, or your pulse is still elevated an hour later, or your friends nicknamed you Insane Gym Demon and even strangers know to avoid making eye contact in the weight room, you can justify picking 11, the highest number, as your intensity factor. If you do a mix of intensities, pick 10. And if you're recovering from an injury or otherwise training at a more casual level, go with 9.

So if you average 5 weekly training hours and give yourself a 10 for your intensity factor, your *activity multiplier* would be: 5 + 10 = 15.

STEP 3: Multiply your activity multiplier by your TBW.

With a TBW of 170, this is your formula: 170 × 15 = 2,550 daily calories.

The Greyhound Formula:
TBW x (11 – 13 + average total weekly training hours)

If you're younger, leaner, have a lot of nervous energy, and struggle to gain weight, you probably have a high level of NEAT. You're what Alan calls a metabolic greyhound. (Tiebreaker question: Can you fit into your girlfriend's jeans?) For you, Alan starts with a higher range of intensity factors to accommodate the calories you burn without trying.

For this example, let's say your TBW is 190 pounds, you work out 4 hours a week on average, and you give yourself a middle-of-the-scale training intensity of 12. Here's how the formula looks.

$$190 \times (12 + 4) = 3{,}040 \text{ daily calories}$$

How to Calculate Macronutrients

Protein

This one's easy: Protein has 4 calories per gram, and you want 1 gram of protein per pound of TBW. Let's assume a TBW of 180: $180 \times 4 = 720$ calories from protein.

Fat

This step is a bit trickier, since there's a range of 0.4 to 0.7 gram per pound of TBW. Some of us feel better with less fat and more carbs, and some of us do better with fewer carbs, which means more fat. Either approach can work. Let's say you pick 0.5, and your TBW is still 180 pounds. Since a gram of fat has 9 calories, this is your formula: $180 \times 0.5 = 90$; $90 \times 9 = 810$ calories from fat.

Carbohydrates

Whatever we have left after calculating protein and fat is your allotment of carbs. We've already included 720 calories from protein and 810 calories from fat, for a total of 1,530 calories. Let's say you calculated a daily requirement of 2,700 calories to hit your TBW of 180 pounds: $2{,}700 - 1{,}530 = 1{,}170$ calories from carbs. And carbs average 4 calories per gram, so: $1{,}170 \div 4 = 292$ grams of carbs.

Keys to Success

The calculations themselves, as you see, aren't difficult. The most important parts are the assumptions behind the calculations.

▶ Estimating your current body-fat percentage

▶ Choosing a realistic body-weight target based on an attainable body-fat percentage

- ▶ Honestly assessing your average training volume and intensity of effort

- ▶ Choosing whether you prefer more fat, more carbs, or a balance of the two

- ▶ Not screwing up basic fourth-grade math

Now let's see how it works for several archetypal guys.

Lean Muscle Diet Case Studies

CASE STUDY #1: DESKBOUND DAN

CURRENT WEIGHT	240 pounds
BODY FAT	30% (obese)
TRAINING STATUS	Beginner
WEEKLY HOURS OF TRAINING	2
INTENSITY OF EFFORT	Moderate
GOAL	Weight loss

As a beginner with a high body-fat percentage, Dan can realistically plan to lose 24 pounds, which is 10 percent of his current weight. That means his TBW is 216 pounds. Since he's sedentary most of the time, we're going to use Alan's Standard Formula, which gives him an activity adjustment of 10 for his moderate intensity level. Add his 2 weekly training hours and we get an activity multiplier of 12. Here's how the math looks: 216 × 12 = 2,592 daily calories.

Macronutrients

As noted, Dan is sedentary most of the time, and he's obese according to both his BMI and his body-fat percentage. So Alan assumes he has a low carbohydrate tolerance, which means he'll get more calories from fat and fewer from carbs.

Protein: 216 grams x 4 = 864 calories

Fat: 216 x 0.6 = 130 grams; 130 x 9 = 1,170 calories

Carbs: 864 calories from protein + 1,170 calories from fat = 2,034 calories

2,592 total calories − 2,034 = 558 calories from carbs

558 ÷ 4 = 139 grams (rounded down)

Now, if 139 grams of carbs—just over 20 percent of his daily calories—seems scary-low to Dan, he can always change the balance. But in the context of popular low-carb diets, 20 percent isn't especially restrictive. It means cutting way back on pizza, sandwiches, pasta, and breakfast cereal, but it leaves room for fruit, nuts, and vegetables. Compare that to the Atkins Diet, which allows just 20 *grams* of carbs in the induction phase, or one medium-size apple.

CASE STUDY #2: SKINNY-FAT STAN

CURRENT WEIGHT	160 pounds
BODY FAT	25% (borderline obese)
TRAINING STATUS	Beginner
WEEKLY HOURS OF TRAINING	4
INTENSITY OF EFFORT	Moderate
GOAL	Simultaneous fat loss and muscle gain

Stan is a victim of the information age: He was in the first generation of students whose physical education was sacrificed for high-stakes testing, and the pressure to perform followed him through college and his first job. The result is a bright, ambitious young man who couldn't beat his own grandmother in arm wrestling. She may actually have more lean tissue than he does.

But here's the good news: As someone who's never done a progressive training program, he's primed for a "culk": simultaneous cutting and bulking. His goal in the next 6 months is to gain 12 pounds of muscle (2 pounds a month), and he should be able to shed an equal amount of fat. This is classic *body recomposition,* a phrase coined by 1990s bodybuilding guru Dan Duchaine.

Although he's not doing any formal program now, he's committed to 4 hours a week of moderately intense training—3 hours in the weight room and an hour of cycling.

You probably think we're going to use Alan's Standard Formula to determine his daily diet. That's what I figured as well. But Alan says the goal of building muscle requires the Greyhound Formula. So his activity adjustment is 12 (for moderate intensity). We'll add 4 (for weekly training hours), giving him an activity multiplier of 16. His TBW is 160 pounds, so: 160 × 16 = 2,560 daily calories.

Macronutrients

Because Stan, like Dan, is sedentary throughout the day, Alan assumes he'll do better with fewer carbs and more fat. So we'll use the same part of the range, giving him 0.6 gram of fat per pound of TBW.

Protein: 160 grams x 4 = 640 calories

Fat: 160 x 0.6 = 96 grams; 96 x 9 = 864 calories

Carbs: 640 calories from protein + 864 calories from fat = 1,504 calories

2,560 total calories − 1,504 = 1,056 calories from carbs

1,056 ÷ 4 = 264 grams

Stan starts the Lean Muscle Plan with 25 percent body fat, which is 40 pounds' worth. If he successfully loses 12 pounds of fat in the next 6 months, he'll finish with 28. If he also builds 12 pounds of muscle, he'll weigh the same 160 pounds, but with 17.5 percent body fat.

Stop for a moment and think about how different he'll look by the end of those 25 weeks. His shoulders will be wider; his chest, back, and arms will be thicker; his legs will have better shape and more pronounced muscle definition; and his waist will be smaller, making all the other changes seem even more impressive. He'll be much, much stronger, and he'll feel a lot more athletic than he does now. He may even start to move like an athlete, without even thinking about it.

CASE STUDY #3: BROTACULAR BOB

CURRENT WEIGHT	190 pounds
BODY FAT	20% (overweight)
TRAINING STATUS	Intermediate
WEEKLY HOURS OF TRAINING	4.5
INTENSITY OF EFFORT	Moderate
GOAL	Fat loss and muscle maintenance

Bob has trained consistently for several years and gained a lot of muscle and strength. He also gets a lot of exercise in an average week: 3 hours in the weight room and an hour and a half of surfing. He's well past the "newbie gains" that Deskbound Dan and Skinny-Fat Stan can count on. In fact, he never passes up a chance to show off his guns in the gym or at the beach. His goal is to lose 10 pounds of fat, giving him a TBW of 180 pounds.

We're going to use Alan's Standard Formula, as we did with Dan. But because Bob trains more, he gets a higher activity multiplier of 14.5: 10 for a moderate overall effort, and 4.5 for total training hours: $180 \times 14.5 = 2,610$ daily calories.

Macronutrients

Because Bob has always been active, Alan assumes he has a decent carb tolerance. Therefore, he'll get more of his energy from carbohydrates than fat.

Protein: 180 grams x 4 = 720 calories

Fat: 180 x 0.5 = 90 grams; 90 x 9 = 810 calories

Carbs: 720 calories from protein + 810 calories from fat = 1,530 calories

2,610 total calories − 1,530 = 1,080 calories from carbs

1,080 ÷ 4 = 270 grams

CASE STUDY #4: BULKING BARRY

CURRENT WEIGHT	160 pounds
BODY FAT	10% (lean)
TRAINING STATUS	Borderline advanced
WEEKLY HOURS OF TRAINING	6
INTENSITY OF EFFORT	High
GOAL	Muscle gain

Barry was born lean and athletic, and even now he has the energy level of 10-year-old twins with ADHD. So, naturally, he wants nothing more than to bulk up. Which is a challenge, given that he trains hard 6 days a week—3 brutal hours a week in the gym (where his intensity motivates 10 percent of the members and scares the other 90 percent), and another 3 hours in his dojo (where even the instructors fake injuries to avoid sparring with him).

To help Barry reach his TBW of 170 pounds, we're going to need Alan's Greyhound Formula, and we're going to use the maximum activity multipliers: 13 (for his intensity level) + 6 (for his weekly training hours). Here's what he needs to eat every day: 170 × 19 = 3,230 daily calories.

Macronutrients

Thanks to his crazy-fast metabolism and crazy-tough training, Barry has better carb tolerance than Buddy the Elf. But unlike Buddy, he's never had much of a sweet tooth, and actually prefers a higher-fat diet. So he'll get 0.6 gram of fat per pound of TBW, which is near the top of the scale.

Protein: 170 grams x 4 = 680 calories

Fat: 170 x 0.6 = 102 grams; 102 x 9 = 918 calories

Carbs: 680 calories from protein + 918 calories from fat = 1,598 calories

3,230 total calories − 1,598 = 1,632 calories from carbs

1,632 ÷ 4 = 408 grams

NONLINEAR CARBOHYDRATE CONSUMPTION

HOP ON THE CARB CYCLE

Talk to people who succeed on a low-carb diet, and you'll get a range of responses. Some feel they've been liberated from chronic, pointless overeating, where one meal just made them hungrier for the next. Others describe it like a famine they survived. Cut off from quick and dependable sources of energy, their mood and workouts both suffer through the transition. The first group thinks they've seen the light; the second group feels trapped in a cage.

The second group, as it happens, includes a lot of people who train hard and struggle to do so without their traditional pre- and postworkout carbs. That's why nutritionists like Alan turn to *nonlinear carbohydrate allotments*: more carbs on training days, fewer on the days in between workouts. You may have heard it referred to as *carb cycling.* Same idea.

Here's the most common way to use it.

Multiply your daily carb quota by 2. You'll have this double ration twice a week. You can pick any 2 days, but it's probably best to do this on Monday and Wednesday, or whenever you do Workout 1 and Workout 2 of the Lean Muscle Plan. (Those are the heaviest workouts, as you'll see in Part Three.) Now multiply your original quota by 0.6, and have that the other 5 days.

Let's say your goal is to lose weight, and you've calculated a measly allotment of 200 carb grams per day. Two days a week, you'll have 400 grams; the other 5 days, you'll have 120 grams.

That's by no means the only way to cycle your carbs, as you can see in Alan's graph.

THE ARAGON NONLINEAR DIETING GRID

AVERAGE DAILY TARGET	x 1.5	x 2	x 2.5	x 3	x 3.5	x 4
1 CARB-UP PER WEEK	0.91	0.83	0.75	0.66	0.58	0.5
2 CARB-UPS PER WEEK	0.8	0.6	0.4	0.2	0	N/A
3 CARB-UPS PER WEEK	0.62	0.25	N/A	N/A	N/A	N/A
4 CARB-UPS PER WEEK	0.33	N/A	N/A	N/A	N/A	N/A

The vertical axis gives you the choice of 1, 2, 3, or 4 days a week with more carbs than your plan allows. The horizontal axis allows you to increase your carb intake on your high-carbs days by any multiple from 1.5 to 4. If you really do want to have a day with four times your normal carbohydrate allotment, it can only be 1 day a week; the other 6 days you get a mere 50 percent of your planned intake. Conversely, if you want to increase carbs by just 50 percent, you can do that four times a week, and have a third of your normal carbs the other 3 days.

The math at those extremes gets pretty complicated, which is why carb cycling is usually limited to 2 or 3 high-carb days. And it's not at all necessary. Most of us are best off going with the simplest option, which is eating the same amount of all three macronutrients every day of the week. Alan only gets into nonlinear carb intakes with clients who struggle to restrict their favorite energy foods every single day.

CHAPTER 6:

THE ONE WITH ALL THE FOOD

HESE FOOD LISTS are categorized according to Alan's mnemonic device, which was introduced in Chapter 2: "Meg's fabulous figure stopped missing fries." As you may recall, the first two letters of each word are also the first two letters of each food group.

- ▶ Meat and other protein-rich foods
- ▶ Fat-rich foods
- ▶ Fibrous vegetables
- ▶ Starchy foods
- ▶ Milk and other dairy products
- ▶ Fruits

A few notes before we get to the lists.

Alan did his best to choose serving sizes that represent what a guy would actually sit down and eat at a meal. It might be slightly more or less than you would choose for yourself. He also used multiple databases to get the numbers you see here. This is, alas, an inexact science, for two reasons. The databases don't all agree with each other, and they did some rounding to get to the numbers they use. Alan then did his own rounding when necessary to avoid endless strings of decimals. This happens with both calorie counts for a whole food and the grams of each component part of the food—the protein, fat, carbohydrates, and the subcategories of each of those macronutrients.

But Alan emphasizes that the numbers are close enough: "Thinking you'll hit everything perfect, right down to the gram, is not only unrealistic, it's an unhealthy way to approach things."

Meat and Other Protein-Rich Foods

Categorizing foods is a messy process. No whole food is all one thing. Protein-rich foods from animals have fat. It could be a little, a lot, or something in between. Whatever it is, you have to account for it. Plant-based protein sources generally have less protein per serving, and with more carbs. Again, you have to account for that.

Then there are the crossover categories. Cheese, for example, is obviously made from milk. But it's also a source of high-quality protein. So Alan includes it in both sections. Same with beans and nuts: Since they check multiple boxes in your diet (protein, starchy carbs, and/or fat), he includes them in multiple charts.

To make it (slightly) easier for you, Alan has six charts in this category, three each for animal and vegetable protein sources: very lean, lean to moderate fat, and high fat.

Most readers will need 4 to 7 servings per day from this group to reach their daily protein targets, assuming each serving has 20 to 30 grams of protein. If you're a vegetarian, you'll probably need 5 to 9 daily servings from those choices.

On all the charts, "cal" is short for calories, and everything else—like protein and fat—is in grams. You'll see that Alan also lists fiber grams for the vegetable sources.

ANIMAL PROTEIN: VERY LEAN

FOOD	SERVING SIZE	CAL	PROTEIN	CARBS	FAT	LEUCINE
BEEF, EYE OF ROUND, FAT TRIMMED OFF, ROASTED	3.5 oz (100 g)	162	29.3	0	4.1	2.3
BEEF, GROUND, 95% LEAN	3.5 oz (100 g)	171	26.3	0	6.5	2.0
BEEF, TOP SIRLOIN, FAT TRIMMED OFF, BROILED	3.5 oz (100 g)	177	30.8	0	5.0	2.5
BISON (BUFFALO), ROASTED	3.5 oz (100 g)	143	28.4	0	2.4	2.2
CANADIAN BACON, COOKED	3.5 oz (100 g)	185	24.2	1.3	8.4	1.7
CARP	3.5 oz (100 g)	162	22.9	0	7.2	1.8
CASEIN PROTEIN POWDER, ELITE CASEIN BY DYMATIZE	1 scoop (32 g)	120	24.0	5	1.0	2.0
CHANNEL CATFISH	3.5 oz (100 g)	105	18.5	0	2.8	1.5
CHEESE, CHEDDAR, FAT FREE	2 slices (60 g)	90	18.0	4.0	0	1.4
CHEESE, COTTAGE, 1% MILK FAT	1 cup (227 g)	163	28.0	6.1	2.3	2.8
CHEESE, COTTAGE, FAT FREE	1 cup (145 g)	104	15.0	9.7	0.4	1.5
CHEESE, MOZZARELLA, FAT FREE	2 oz (57 g)	90	18.0	4.0	0	1.4
CHEESE, LOW FAT, CHEDDAR OR COLBY	⅔ cup, shredded (75 g)	129	18.1	1.5	5.2	1.8
CHICKEN BREAST (MEAT ONLY), ROASTED	3.5 oz (100 g)	165	31.0	0	3.6	2.3
CHICKEN BREAST (MEAT AND SKIN), ROASTED	3.5 oz (100 g)	197	29.8	0	7.8	2.2
CLAM	3.5 oz (100 g)	148	25.5	5.1	1.9	1.8

(continued)

ANIMAL PROTEIN: VERY LEAN *(cont.)*

FOOD	SERVING SIZE	CAL	PROTEIN	CARBS	FAT	LEUCINE
COD, ATLANTIC	3.5 oz (100 g)	105	22.8	0	0.9	1.8
CRAB, ALASKA KING, COOKED	1 leg, 4.8 oz (136 g)	130	25.9	0	2.1	2.0
EGG PROTEIN POWDER (WHITES), GOLD STANDARD 100% EGG BY OPTIMUM NUTRITION	1 scoop (35 g)	130	24.0	5.0	1.0	2.0
EGG WHITES, RAW	1 cup or 8–12 whites (243 g)	117	26.5	1.8	0.4	2.5
ELK, ROUND, BROILED	3.5 oz (100 g)	156	30.9	0	2.6	2.3
EMU, FULL RUMP, BROILED	3.5 oz (100 g)	168	33.7	0	2.7	1.8
FLATFISH (FLOUNDER AND SOLE)	3.5 oz (100 g)	117	24.2	0	1.5	2.0
GOAT, ROASTED	3.5 oz (100 g)	143	27.1	0	3	2.3
HADDOCK	3.5 oz (100 g)	112	24.2	0	0.9	2.0
HAM, EXTRA LEAN	3.5 oz (100 g)	107	18.8	0.7	2.6	1.5
LOBSTER	3.5 oz (100 g)	98	20.5	1.3	0.6	1.6
ORANGE ROUGHY	3.5 oz (100 g)	105	22.6	0	0.9	1.8
OSTRICH, TOP LOIN	3.5 oz (100 g)	155	28.1	0	3.9	2.3
OYSTER, PACIFIC, RAW	5 medium (250 g)	202	23.5	12.5	5.5	1.7
PASTRAMI	3.5 oz (100 g)	146	21.8	0.1	5.8	1.7
PIKE, WALLEYE	3.5 oz (100 g)	119	24.5	0	1.6	2.0

FOOD	SERVING SIZE	CAL	PROTEIN	CARBS	FAT	LEUCINE
POLLOCK, WALLEYE	3.5 oz (100 g)	113	23.5	0	1.1	1.9
PORK, TENDERLOIN, ROASTED	3.5 oz (100 g)	143	26.2	0	3.5	2.2
SALMON, CANNED	3.5 oz (100 g)	139	19.8	0	6.1	1.6
SALMON, SMOKED (LOX)	3.5 oz (100 g)	117	18.3	0	4.3	1.5
SEA BASS	3.5 oz (100 g)	124	23.6	0	2.6	1.9
SHRIMP, COOKED	3.5 oz (100 g)	99	20.9	0	1.1	1.7
SNAPPER	3.5 oz (100 g)	128	26.3	0	1.7	2.1
SWORDFISH	3.5 oz (100 g)	155	25.4	0	5.1	2.1
TILAPIA	3.5 oz (100 g)	128	26.1	0	2.7	2.0
TROUT, RAINBOW	3.5 oz (100 g)	169	24.3	0	7.2	1.9
TUNA, LIGHT, CANNED IN WATER, DRAINED	3.5 oz (100 g)	116	25.5	0	0.8	2.1
TUNA, YELLOWFIN	3.5 oz (100 g)	139	30.0	0	1.2	2.4
TURKEY BREAST, MEAT ONLY, ROASTED	3.5 oz (100 g)	135	30.1	0	0.7	2.4
VEAL, LOIN, BRAISED	3.5 oz (100 g)	226	33.6	0	9.2	2.7
VENISON (DEER), SHOULDER CLOD	3.5 oz (100 g)	191	36.3	0	3.9	2.7
WHEY PROTEIN POWDER, ELITE WHEY BY DYMATIZE	1 scoop (34.9 g)	130	25.0	3.0	1.5	3.0
WHITEFISH	3.5 oz (100 g)	172	24.5	0	7.5	2.0
YOGURT, GREEK, FAT FREE	1 cup (224 g)	120	20.0	9.0	0	1.6

(continued)

ANIMAL PROTEIN: LEAN TO MODERATE FAT

FOOD	SERVING SIZE	CAL	PROTEIN	CARBS	FAT	LEUCINE
ANCHOVY, EUROPEAN, CANNED IN OIL	3.5 oz (100 g)	210	28.9	0	9.7	2.3
BEEF, CORNED, BRISKET	3.5 oz (100 g)	251	18.2	0	19.0	1.4
BEEF, GROUND SIRLOIN, 90% LEAN	3.5 oz (100 g)	214	26.6	0	11.1	2.0
BEEF, GROUND, 85% LEAN	3.5 oz (100 g)	250	25.9	0	15.5	2.0
BEEF, PRIME RIB, ROASTED	3.5 oz (100 g)	266	26.0	0	17.0	2.0
BEEF, SHORTRIBS, BRAISED	3.5 oz (100 g)	295	30.8	0	18.1	2.4
CHEESE, FETA, REDUCED FAT	⅔ cup (150 g)	206	21.0	0	13.0	1.7
CHEESE, MOZZARELLA, REDUCED FAT	3.5 oz (100 g)	254	24.3	2.8	15.9	2.4
CHEESE, RICOTTA, REDUCED FAT	⅔ cup (162 g)	224	18.5	8.3	12.9	2.0
CHICKEN LEG, MEAT AND SKIN, ROASTED	3.5 oz (100 g)	232	26.0	0	13.5	1.9
CHICKEN THIGH, MEAT ONLY, ROASTED	3.5 oz (100 g)	209	25.9	0	10.9	1.9
CHICKEN WING, MEAT AND SKIN, ROASTED	3.5 oz (100 g)	290	26.9	0	19.5	1.9
DUCK, ROASTED	3.5 oz (100 g)	201	23.5	0	11.2	2.0
EGG, HARD BOILED OR POACHED	3 large (150 g)	232	18.9	1.8	15.9	1.6
HERRING, ATLANTIC, KIPPERED	3.5 oz (100 g)	217	24.6	0	12.4	2.0
LAMB FORESHANK, FAT TRIMMED, BRAISED	3.5 oz (100 g)	243	28.4	0	13.5	2.2
LAMB, GROUND	3.5 oz (100 g)	283	24.7	0	19.7	1.9
PORK CHOP, BONE-IN, BRAISED	3.5 oz (100 g)	250	26.7	0	15.1	2.1

FOOD	SERVING SIZE	CAL	PROTEIN	CARBS	FAT	LEUCINE
SAUSAGE, BEEF/CHICKEN/PORK, SMOKED	3.5 oz (100 g)	216	13.6	8.1	14.3	1.0
SALMON, ATLANTIC	3.5 oz (100 g)	206	22.1	0	12.3	1.8
SARDINE, PACIFIC, CANNED IN TOMATO SAUCE	3.5 oz (100 g)	186	20.9	0.7	10.5	1.4
TURKEY, GROUND	3.5 oz (100 g)	235	27.4	0	13.1	2.1
TURKEY SAUSAGE	3.5 oz (100 g)	196	23.9	0	10.4	1.7

ANIMAL PROTEIN: HIGH FAT

FOOD	SERVING SIZE	CAL	PROTEIN	CARBS	FAT	LEUCINE
BACON	2 oz (57 g)	298	21.4	0.8	22.6	1.7
BEEF TONGUE	3.5 oz (100 g)	284	19.3	0	22.3	2.0
CHEESE, AMERICAN	3 oz (85 g)	315	18.6	1.2	26.4	1.6
CHEESE, BLUE	3 oz (85 g)	297	18.0	2.1	24.0	1.6
CHEESE, CHEDDAR	⅔ cup, (75 g)	300	18.5	0.9	24.8	1.6
CHEESE, FETA	1 cup (150 g)	396	21.3	0	31.9	1.7
CHEESE, GOAT, HARD	3 oz (85 g)	381	25.5	1.8	30.0	2.1
CHEESE, MONTEREY JACK	3 oz (85 g)	300	21.0	1.0	27.0	1.6
CHEESE, SWISS	3 oz (85 g)	318	22.5	4.5	23.4	1.8
EGG, FRIED	3 large (138 g)	271	18.9	1.2	21.0	1.6
SAUSAGE, BEEF	3.5 oz (100 g)	332	18.2	0.4	28.0	1.5
SAUSAGE, PORK	3.5 oz (100 g)	339	19.4	0	28.4	1.3

VEGETABLE PROTEIN: VERY LEAN

FOOD	SERVING SIZE	CAL	PROTEIN	CARBS	FAT	LEUCINE	FIBER
BEANS, BLACK	1 cup (172 g)	227	15.2	40.8	0.9	1.2	15.0
BEANS, KIDNEY	1 cup (177 g)	225	15.3	40.4	0.9	1.3	11.3
BEANS, LIMA	1 cup (188 g)	216	14.7	39.3	0.7	1.3	13.2
BEANS, NAVY	1 cup (182 g)	255	15.0	47.8	1.1	1.3	19.1
BEANS, PINTO	1 cup (171 g)	245	15.4	44.8	1.1	1.1	15.4
BEANS, REFRIED, CANNED	1 cup (238 g)	217	12.9	36.3	2.8	1.0	12.1
BEANS, WHITE	1 cup (179 g)	249	17.4	44.9	0.6	1.4	11.3
CHICKPEAS (GAR- BANZO BEANS)	1 cup (164 g)	269	14.5	45.0	4.2	1.0	12.5
COWPEAS (BLACK-EYED)	1 cup (172 g)	200	13.3	35.7	0.9	1.0	11.2
EDAMAME (SOY- BEANS), FROZEN	1 cup (155 g)	189	16.9	15.8	8.1	1.2	8.1
GEMMA PEA PRO- TEIN ISOLATE	1 scoop (30 g)	120	24.6	1.2	1.8	2.4	1.2
HEMP PROTEIN POWDER	1 oz (28 g)	113	12.6	7.0	3.4	1	4.8
LENTILS	1 cup (198 g)	230	17.9	39.9	0.8	1.3	15.6
PEAS, GREEN	1.5 cups (240 g)	187	12.3	34.2	0.6	0.7	13.2
PEAS, SPLIT	1 cup (196 g)	231	16.3	41.4	0.8	1.2	16.3
SOY MILK, SILK BRAND	2 cups (486 g)	200	14.0	16.0	8.0	1.1	1.0
SOY PROTEIN POWDER, OPTIMUM NUTRI- TION'S 100% SOY PROTEIN	1 scoop (31.5 g)	120	25.0	2.0	1.5	2.0	0

FOOD	SERVING SIZE	CAL	PROTEIN	CARBS	FAT	LEUCINE	FIBER
VEGETARIAN MEATLOAF	3.5 oz (100 g)	197	21.0	8.0	9.0	1.7	4.6
VEGGIE OR SOY BURGERS	2 patties (140 g total)	248	22.0	20.0	8.8	1.9	6.8
WHEAT GERM, TOASTED	½ cup (56 g)	216	16.4	28.0	6.0	1.1	8.5

VEGETABLE PROTEIN: LEAN TO MODERATE FAT

FOOD	SERVING SIZE	CAL	PROTEIN	CARBS	FAT	LEUCINE	FIBER
FALAFEL	3.5 oz (100 g)	333	13.3	31.8	17.8	0.9	4.0
HUMMUS	⅔ cup (162 g)	269	12.8	23.2	15.6	0.9	6.5
SOYBEANS, ROASTED	⅓ cup (57 g)	256	22.4	18.5	12.2	1.8	4.6
TEMPEH, COOKED	3.5 oz (100 g)	196	18.2	9.4	11.4	1.4	9.0
TOFU, FIRM (NIGARI)	1 cup (252 g)	176	20.6	4.2	10.6	1.8	2.2

VEGETABLE PROTEIN: HIGH FAT

FOOD	SERVING SIZE	CAL	PROTEIN	CARBS	FAT	LEUCINE	FIBER
ALMONDS	⅔ cup, whole (94 g)	542	20.0	20.5	46.9	1.4	11.5
BRAZIL NUTS	⅔ cup, whole (88 g)	575	12.5	10.8	58.3	1.0	6.6
CASHEWS	⅔ cup, whole (100 g)	553	13.9	29.6	41.9	1.2	2.7
CHIA SEEDS, WHOLE	⅔ cup (100 g)	490	15.6	43.8	30.8	1.3	37.7
FLAXSEEDS, WHOLE	⅔ cup (111 g)	592	20.3	32.0	46.7	1.4	30.3

(continued)

VEGETABLE PROTEIN: HIGH FAT *(cont.)*

FOOD	SERVING SIZE	CAL	PROTEIN	CARBS	FAT	LEUCINE	FIBER
HAZELNUTS	⅔ cup (76 g)	477	11.3	12.7	46.1	0.8	7.4
PEANUTS	⅔ cup (96 g)	564	22.8	20.7	47.8	1.5	7.7
PISTACHIOS	⅔ cup (81 g)	463	17.4	22.4	37.3	1.3	8.4
PUMPKIN OR SQUASH SEEDS, UNSHELLED	⅔ cup (91 g)	493	22.4	16.2	41.8	1.9	3.6
SESAME SEEDS, WHOLE	⅔ cup (100 g)	565	17.0	25.7	48	1.3	14.0
SUNFLOWER SEEDS, UNSHELLED	1 cup (46 g)	269	9.6	9.2	23.7	0.8	4.0
TAHINI	¼ cup (60 g)	357	10.2	12.7	32.2	0.7	5.6
WALNUTS	⅔ cup (77 g)	505	11.7	10.6	50.4	0.9	5.1

Fat-Rich Foods

All fat-rich foods have a mix of fatty acids. That applies to the higher-fat foods in the previous category as well as these. But they're typically higher in one type of fat—saturated (SFA), monounsaturated (MUFA), or polyunsaturated (PUFA)—which is why Alan groups them that way.

Some of the choices are listed by teaspoon (tsp) or tablespoon (Tbsp). Three teaspoons equal 1 tablespoon. Four tablespoons equal ¼ cup.

Finally, you may be surprised by where some foods appear. Bacon grease and lard, for example, are traditionally considered high in saturated fats. But they actually have more monounsaturated fat, which is why Alan listed them in that category.

HIGHEST IN SATURATED FAT

FOOD	SERVING SIZE	CAL	PROTEIN	CARBS	FAT	SFA	MUFA	PUFA
BUTTER	1 pat (5 g)	36	0	0	4.1	2.6	1.1	0.2
COCONUT MILK, RAW	1 Tbsp (15 g)	35	0.3	0.8	3.6	3.2	0.2	0
COCONUT, UNSWEET-ENED, SHREDDED	3 Tbsp (15 g)	100	1.0	4.0	10.0	9.0	0.5	0.3
CREAM CHEESE	1 Tbsp (14 g)	50	0.9	0.6	5.0	2.8	1.2	0.2
CREAM, HALF & HALF	¼ cup (60 g)	79	1.8	2.6	7.0	4.3	2.0	0.2
CREAM, HEAVY WHIPPING	¼ cup (30 g)	103	0.6	0.8	11.1	6.9	3.2	0.4
CREAM, SOUR	2 Tbsp (24 g)	46	0.4	0.8	4.8	2.8	1.2	0.2
OIL, COCONUT	1 tsp (4.5 g)	38	0	0	4.5	3.9	0.3	0.1
OIL, PALM	1 tsp (4.5 g)	40	0	0	4.5	2.2	1.7	0.4

HIGHEST IN MONOUNSATURATED FAT

FOOD	SERVING SIZE	CAL	PROTEIN	CARBS	FAT	SFA	MUFA	PUFA
ALMONDS	1 oz or slightly less than ¼ cup (28 g)	162	6.0	6.1	14.0	1.1	8.7	3.4
AVOCADO	½ large (201 g)	161	2.0	8.9	14.7	2.1	9.9	1.8
BACON GREASE	1 tsp (4 g)	38	0	0	4.2	1.7	1.9	0.5
BRAZIL NUTS	1 oz (28 g)	184	4.0	3.4	18.6	4.2	6.9	5.8

(continued)

HIGHEST IN MONUNSATURATED FAT *(cont.)*

FOOD	SERVING SIZE	CAL	PROTEIN	CARBS	FAT	SFA	MUFA	PUFA
BUTTER, ALMOND	1 Tbsp (16 g)	101	2.4	3.4	9.5	0.9	6.1	2.0
BUTTER, CASHEW	1 Tbsp (16 g)	94	2.8	4.4	7.9	1.6	4.7	1.3
BUTTER, PEANUT	1 Tbsp (16 g)	94	4.0	3.2	8.0	1.7	3.8	2.2
CASHEWS	1 oz or slightly less than ¼ cup (28 g)	155	5.1	9.2	12.3	2.2	6.7	2.2
HAZELNUTS	1 oz or slightly less than ¼ cup (28 g)	176	4.2	4.7	17.0	1.3	12.8	2.2
LARD	1 Tbsp (13 g)	115	0	0	12.8	5.0	5.8	1.4
MACADAMIA NUTS	1 oz or slightly less than ¼ cup (28 g)	201	2.2	4.0	21.2	3.4	16.5	0.4
OIL, CANOLA	1 tsp (4.5 g)	40	0	0	4.5	0.3	2.8	1.3
OIL, COD LIVER	1 tsp (4.5 g)	41	0	0	4.5	1.0	2.1	1.0
OIL, OLIVE	1 tsp (4.5 g)	40	0	0	4.5	0.6	3.3	0.5
OIL, PEANUT	1 tsp (4.5 g)	40	0	0	4.5	0.8	2.1	1.4
OIL, SAFFLOWER	1 tsp (4.5 g)	40	0	0	4.5	0.3	3.4	0.6
OIL, SUNFLOWER	1 tsp (4.5 g)	40	0	0	4.5	0.4	2.6	1.3
OLIVES	1 oz or 6–9 whole (28 g)	41	0.3	1.1	4.3	0.6	3.2	0.4

FOOD	SERVING SIZE	CAL	PROTEIN	CARBS	FAT	SFA	MUFA	PUFA
PEANUTS	1 oz or slightly less than ¼ cup (28 g)	164	6.6	6.0	13.9	1.9	6.9	4.4
PECANS	1 oz or slightly less than ¼ cup (28 g)	199	2.7	3.8	20.8	1.8	12.3	5.8
PISTACHIOS	1 oz or slightly less than ¼ cup (28 g)	160	6.0	7.7	12.9	1.6	6.8	3.9

HIGHEST IN POLYUNSATURATED FAT

FOOD	SERVING SIZE	CAL	PROTEIN	CARBS	FAT	SFA	MUFA	PUFA
FISH OIL, MIXED COLD-WATER SPECIES	1 tsp (5 g)	40	0	0	5.0	1.0	1.0	2.0
FISH OIL, SALMON	1 tsp (4.5 g)	41	0	0	4.5	0.9	1.3	1.8
FLAXSEEDS, WHOLE	1 Tbsp (10 g)	55	1.9	3.0	4.3	0.4	0.8	2.9
MAYONNAISE, LIGHT	1 Tbsp (14 g)	48	0.1	1.0	4.8	0.7	1.1	2.8
MAYONNAISE, REGULAR	1 Tbsp (15 g)	90	0.1	0	10.0	1.5	2.5	6.0
OIL, CORN	1 tsp (4.5 g)	40	0	0	4.5	0.6	1.2	2.5
OIL, FLAXSEED	1 tsp (4.5 g)	40	0	0	4.5	0.4	0.9	3.0

(continued)

HIGHEST IN POLYUNSATURATED FAT *(cont.)*

FOOD	SERVING SIZE	CAL	PROTEIN	CARBS	FAT	SFA	MUFA	PUFA
OIL, GRAPESEED	1 tsp (4.5 g)	40	0	0	4.5	0.4	0.7	3.1
OIL, SESAME	1 tsp (4.5 g)	40	0	0	4.5	0.6	1.8	1.9
OIL, SOYBEAN	1 tsp (4.5 g)	40	0	0	4.5	0.7	1.0	2.6
SALAD DRESSING, ITALIAN	1 Tbsp (14 g)	42	0.1	1.5	4.1	0.6	0.9	1.9
SALAD DRESSING, RANCH	1 Tbsp (15 g)	73	0.2	1.0	7.7	1.2	1.7	4.2
WALNUTS	1 oz or slightly less than ¼ cup (28 g)	185	4.3	3.9	18.4	1.7	2.5	13.3

Fibrous Vegetables

It's convenient to call these foods "fibrous" vegetables, mostly to distinguish them from starchy vegetables. But they aren't all high in fiber, as you'll see in the chart. The main thing they have in common is low calories. It would take some work to overeat veggies, which is why diet plans typically put no limit on them.

FOOD	SERVING SIZE	CAL	PROTEIN	CARBS	FAT	FIBER
ARTICHOKE, COOKED	1 medium (120 g)	64	3.5	14.3	0.4	10.3
ASPARAGUS, COOKED	½ cup (90 g)	20	2.2	3.7	0.2	1.8
ASPARAGUS, RAW	7 medium spears (112 g)	23	2.8	3.0	0	2.1

FOOD	SERVING SIZE	CAL	PROTEIN	CARBS	FAT	FIBER
BAMBOO SHOOTS, BOILED	½ cup (120 g)	14	1.8	2.3	0.3	1.2
BEAN SPROUTS, SOYBEAN OR MUNG	1 cup (100 g)	30	3.0	5.9	0.2	1.8
BOK CHOY (CHINESE CABBAGE), BOILED	1 cup shredded (170 g)	20	2.1	11.7	0.3	1.7
BROCCOLI, FLOWER CLUSTERS, RAW	1 cup (71 g)	20	2.1	3.7	0.2	2.3
BROCCOLI, COOKED	1 medium stalk (180 g)	63	4.3	12.9	0.7	5.9
BRUSSELS SPROUTS, BOILED	½ cup (78 g)	28	2.0	5.5	0.4	2.0
CABBAGE, RAW	1 cup chopped (89 g)	22	1.1	5.2	0.1	2.2
CARROTS, RAW	1 medium (61 g)	25	0.6	5.8	0.1	1.7
CARROTS, COOKED	½ cup sliced (78 g)	27	0.6	6.4	0.1	2.3
CAULIFLOWER, RAW	1 cup (100 g)	25	2.0	5.3	0.1	2.5
CAULIFLOWER, COOKED	1 cup (124 g)	29	2.2	5.4	0.6	2.8
CELERY	1 large stalk (64 g)	10	0.4	2.2	0.1	1.0
CHARD, RAW	1 cup (36 g)	7.0	0.6	1.3	0.1	0.6
COLLARD GREENS, BOILED	1 cup chopped (190 g)	49	4.0	9.3	0.7	5.3
GREEN SNAP BEANS	1 cup (110 g)	34	2.0	7.8	0.1	3.7
GREEN STRING BEANS	1 cup (100 g)	31	1.8	7.1	0.1	3.4

(continued)

FIBROUS VEGETABLES *(cont.)*

FOOD	SERVING SIZE	CAL	PROTEIN	CARBS	FAT	FIBER
JICAMA (YAMBEAN), RAW	1 cup sliced (120 g)	46	0.9	10.6	0.1	5.9
KALE, COOKED	1 cup chopped (130 g)	36	2.5	7.3	0.5	2.6
LEEKS, COOKED	1 leek (124 g)	38	1.0	9.4	0.2	1.2
LETTUCE, ICEBERG	2 cups shredded (144 g)	20	1.2	4.6	0.2	1.8
LETTUCE, ROMAINE	2 cups shredded	16	1.2	3.0	0.2	2.0
MUSHROOM, PORTOBELLO, GRILLED	1 piece whole (100 g)	35	4.3	4.9	0.7	2.2
MUSHROOMS, SHII-TAKE, COOKED	½ cup pieces (73 g)	81	2.3	20.9	0.3	3.0
MUSHROOMS, WHITE, RAW	1 cup sliced (70 g)	15	2.2	2.3	0.2	0.7
MUSTARD GREENS, COOKED	1 cup chopped (140 g)	21	3.2	2.9	0.3	2.8
OKRA, BOILED	½ cup sliced (80 g)	18	1.5	3.9	0.2	2.0
ONIONS, RAW	½ cup chopped (80 g)	32	0.9	7.4	0.1	1.4
ONIONS, COOKED	½ cup (105 g)	44	1.4	10.5	0.2	1.5
PEAS, SUGAR SNAP, RAW	1 cup whole (63 g)	26	1.8	4.8	0.1	1.6
PEPPER, HOT CHILE, RED, RAW	1 pepper (45 g)	18	0.8	4.0	0.2	0.7
PEPPER, SWEET BELL, COOKED	1 cup chopped or in strips (135 g)	38	1.2	9.0	0.3	1.6

FOOD	SERVING SIZE	CAL	PROTEIN	CARBS	FAT	FIBER
RADISHES, RAW	1 cup sliced (116)	19	0.8	4.0	0.1	1.9
RUTABAGAS, COOKED	1 cup cubed (170 g)	66	2.2	14.9	0.4	3.1
SPINACH, RAW	2 cups (60 g)	14	1.8	2.2	0.2	1.4
SQUASH, SUMMER (INCLUDING ZUCCHINI), COOKED	1 cup sliced (180 g)	36	1.6	7.8	0.6	2.5
TOMATO, RED, RAW	1 medium whole (123 g)	22	1.1	4.8	0.2	1.5
TOMATO SAUCE	½ cup (122 g)	51	1.6	10.7	0.2	1.8
TURNIPS, COOKED	1 cup cubed (156 g)	34	1.1	7.9	0.1	3.1
TURNIP GREENS, COOKED	1 cup chopped (144 g)	29	1.6	6.3	0.3	5.0
WATER CHESTNUTS, CANNED	½ cup sliced (70 g)	35	0.6	8.6	0	1.8

Starchy Foods

Starches are an easy target for fad diets. It makes some sense, especially when looking at tasty, highly processed, easy-to-overeat grains. But where some see evil, Alan sees nuance. That's why he subdivides them into two categories: grains and grain products, and starchy vegetables. The second category includes legumes (beans, peas, lentils), which are also listed with protein-rich foods. All, he believes, can be eaten in moderation without compromising your goals.

One housekeeping note: Alan includes corn with the grains, even though some regard it as a vegetable (in which case it'd fall into the same category as potatoes and other tubers), or even a fruit. The key is that it's a starch-dominant food; it doesn't matter which category of starch it falls into.

GRAINS AND GRAIN PRODUCTS

FOOD	SERVING SIZE	CAL	PROTEIN	CARBS	FAT	FIBER
BAGEL, PLAIN	1 medium (105 g)	289	11.9	56.1	1.7	2.4
BARLEY, COOKED	1 cup (157 g)	193	3.5	44.3	0.7	6.0
BREAD, NAAN (INDIAN FLATBREAD)	¼ piece with 10-in diameter (44 g)	137	3.7	18.8	5.1	0.7
BREAD, PITA	1 large (60 g)	165	5.5	33.4	0.7	1.3
BREAD, RYE	1 slice (32 g)	83	2.7	15.5	1.1	1.9
BREAD, WHITE	1 slice (30 g)	80	2.3	15.2	1.0	0.7
BREAD, WHOLE WHEAT	1 slice (28 g)	69	3.5	11.6	0.9	1.9
BULGUR, COOKED	1 cup (182 g)	151	5.6	33.8	0.4	8.2
CEREAL, DRY, WHEAT BASED	1 cup (38 g)	120	3.5	30.1	0.9	6.6
CEREAL, DRY, OAT BASED	1 cup (40 g)	150	6.0	27.0	2.5	4.0
CORN, SWEET, YELLOW	1 cup cut (164 g)	177	5.4	41.2	2.1	4.6
CORN ON THE COB	1 medium (103 g)	111	3.4	25.9	1.3	2.9
COUSCOUS, COOKED	1 cup (157 g)	176	5.9	36.5	0.3	2.2
DINNER ROLL	1 roll (28 g)	85	2.4	14.3	2.1	0.9
GRITS, COOKED	1 cup (242 g)	145	3.4	31.5	0.5	0.5
MUESLI WITH DRIED FRUITS AND NUTS	½ cup (42 g)	145	4.1	33.0	2.1	3.2
OATMEAL, ALL TYPES, COOKED	1 cup (234 g)	166	5.9	31.8	3.6	4.0
PASTA, ALL TYPES, COOKED	1 cup	186	6.3	38.4	0.9	1.5
QUINOA, COOKED	1 cup (185 g)	222	8.1	39.4	3.6	5.2
TORTILLA, CORN	1 medium, 6 in (26 g)	58	1.5	12.1	0.7	1.4
TORTILLA, FLOUR	1 medium, 7–8 in (70 g)	144	3.8	23.6	3.6	1.4

FOOD	SERVING SIZE	CAL	PROTEIN	CARBS	FAT	FIBER
RICE, BROWN, MEDIUM GRAIN, COOKED	1 cup (195 g)	218	4.5	45.8	1.6	3.5
RICE, WHITE, LONG GRAIN, COOKED	1 cup (158 g)	205	4.2	44.5	0.4	0.6

STARCHY VEGETABLES

FOOD	SERVING SIZE	CAL	PROTEIN	CARBS	FAT	FIBER
BEANS, BLACK	1 cup (172 g)	227	15.2	40.8	0.9	15.0
BEANS, KIDNEY	1 cup (177 g)	225	15.3	40.4	0.9	11.3
BEANS, LIMA	1 cup (188 g)	216	14.7	39.3	0.7	13.2
BEANS, NAVY	1 cup (182 g)	255	15.0	47.8	1.1	19.1
BEANS, PINTO	1 cup (171 g)	245	15.4	44.8	1.1	15.4
BEANS, REFRIED, CANNED	1 cup (238 g)	217	12.9	36.3	2.8	12.1
BEANS, WHITE	1 cup (179 g)	249	17.4	44.9	0.6	11.3
CASSAVA (YUCCA), COOKED	1 cup, cubed (132 g)	210	1.8	50.1	0.3	2.4
CHICKPEAS (GARBANZO BEANS)	1 cup (164 g)	269	14.5	45	4.2	12.5
COWPEAS (BLACK-EYED)	1 cup (172 g)	200	13.3	35.7	0.9	11.2
EDAMAME (SOYBEANS)	1 cup (155 g)	189	16.9	15.8	8.1	8.1
LENTILS	1 cup (198 g)	230	17.9	39.9	0.8	15.6
PARSNIPS, FRESH, COOKED	1 cup sliced (156 g)	111	2.0	26.6	0.4	5.6
PLANTAINS, COOKED	1 cup, slices (154 g)	179	1.2	48.0	0.3	3.5
POTATO, RUSSET, COOKED	1 medium (173 g)	168	4.5	37.1	0.2	4.0

(continued)

STARCHY VEGETABLES *(cont.)*

FOOD	SERVING SIZE	CAL	PROTEIN	CARBS	FAT	FIBER
POTATO, SWEET, COOKED	1 large (180 g)	162	3.6	37.3	0.3	5.9
PUMPKIN, CANNED	1 cup (245 g)	83	2.7	19.8	0.7	7.1
SQUASH, WINTER, BUTTERNUT, COOKED	1 cup cubed (205 g)	82	1.8	21.5	0.2	3.0
YAMS, COOKED	1 cup cubed (136 g)	158	2.0	37.4	0.2	5.3

Milk and Other Dairy Products

You may recall from Chapter 2 that Alan made a strong argument in favor of milk and other dairy products for those who can tolerate them—that is, those who aren't allergic or lactose-intolerant. That includes the majority of people in North America and Europe.

A generation ago this went without saying; most of us grew up with milk presented as a key part of a healthy diet. Today, while we have substantial research supporting its health benefits (some, but not all, sponsored by the deep-pocketed dairy industry), we have some very loud voices arguing against dairy. It may be the only thing paleo dieters and vegans agree on.

That's why it's important to reiterate its value for your muscles and bones (and why Alan repeats some foods that were included in the protein section). Cow's milk has more protein and calcium per calorie than any other known and naturally occurring food.

For those who are allergic or lactose-intolerant, or vegan, or otherwise dairy-averse, Alan includes soy and almond milk here, the latter reluctantly, since it has too little protein to be considered a true dairy substitute.

FOOD	SERVING SIZE	CAL	PROTEIN	CARBS	FAT	CALCIUM (MG)
ALMOND MILK, CALCIUM FORTIFIED	1 cup	60	1.0	8.0	2.5	300
BUTTERMILK, LOW FAT	1 cup (245 g)	98	8.1	11.7	2.2	284
BUTTERMILK, REDUCED FAT	1 cup (245 g)	137	10.0	13.0	4.9	350
CHEESE, CHEDDAR	1 oz or 1 slice (28 g)	113	7.0	0.4	9.3	202
CHEESE, LOW-FAT CHEDDAR OR COLBY	1 oz or 1 slice (28 g)	48	6.8	0.5	2.0	116
CHEESE, MOZZARELLA, REDUCED FAT	1 oz, 1 slice, or about ⅛ cup (28 g)	71	6.8	0.8	4.5	219
CHOCOLATE MILK, LOW FAT	1 cup (250 g)	157	8.1	26.1	2.5	288
COW'S MILK, FAT FREE	1 cup (245 g)	91	8.7	12.3	0.6	316
COW'S MILK, 1% MILK FAT	1 cup (245 g)	105	8.5	12.2	2.4	314
COW'S MILK, 2% MILK FAT	1 cup (245 g)	137	9.7	13.5	4.9	350
COW'S MILK, 3.25% MILK FAT	1 cup (244 g)	146	7.9	12.8	7.9	276
GOAT'S MILK, WHOLE	1 cup (244 g)	168	8.7	10.9	10.1	327
KEFIR (FERMENTED COW'S MILK)	1 cup (245 g)	120	14.0	11.0	2.5	300
LACTAID (LACTOSE-FREE MILK)	1 cup (240 g)	130	7.9	13.0	5.0	300
SOY MILK, LOW FAT, CALCIUM FORTIFIED	1 cup (243 g)	100	4.0	17.5	1.5	199
YOGURT, FRUIT, FAT FREE	1 container, 6 oz (170 g)	161	7.5	32.3	0.3	258
YOGURT, GREEK, FAT FREE	1 cup (224 g)	120	20.0	9.0	0	250

(continued)

MILK AND OTHER DAIRY PRODUCTS *(cont.)*

FOOD	SERVING SIZE	CAL	PROTEIN	CARBS	FAT	CALCIUM (MG)
YOGURT, PLAIN, LOW FAT	1 cup (245 g)	154	12.9	17.2	3.8	448
YOGURT, PLAIN, FAT FREE	1 cup (245 g)	137	14.0	18.8	0.4	488
YOGURT, PLAIN, FULL FAT	1 cup (245 g)	149	8.5	11.4	8.0	296

Fruits

And we finish with foods that (almost) everyone agrees are a part of a healthy diet. (Super-low-carb dieters, naturally, think they have too many carbs.) One fruit you won't find here: avocados. They're listed with the fat-rich foods for the obvious reason that an avocado has about 30 grams of fat. But it also has 10 grams of fiber, making it one of the most filling and nutrient-dense foods you can consume.

FOOD	SERVING SIZE	CAL	PROTEIN	CARBS	FAT	FIBER
APPLE, FRESH	1 medium (182 g)	95	0.5	25.1	0.3	4.4
APPLE, DRIED	½ cup (43 g)	104	0.8	28.4	0.1	3.7
APPLESAUCE, UNSWEETENED	1 cup (244 g)	102	0.4	27.5	0.2	2.7
APRICOT, FRESH	3 whole (100 g)	48	1.4	11.2	0.4	2.0
APRICOT, DRIED	⅓ cup (43 g)	104	1.5	27.1	0.2	3.1
BANANA	1 medium (118 g)	105	1.3	27.0	0.4	3.1
BLUEBERRIES, FRESH	1 cup (148 g)	84	1.1	21.4	0.5	3.6
BLUEBERRIES, DRIED	⅓ cup (40 g)	130	1.0	31.0	0	3.0
CANTALOUPE	1.5 cups, cubes (160 g)	81	1.9	21.1	0.4	2.1
CHERRIES, FRESH	1 cup (138 g)	87	1.5	22.1	0.3	2.9
CHERRIES, DRIED	¼ cup (40 g)	136	1.0	32.0	0	1.0

FOOD	SERVING SIZE	CAL	PROTEIN	CARBS	FAT	FIBER
CRANBERRIES, DRIED	⅓ cup (40 g)	123	0	32.9	0.5	2.3
DATES, MEDJOOL	2–3 dates, pitted (48 g)	110	1.0	29.0	0	2.0
FIGS, FRESH	2 large (128 g)	94	1.0	24.6	0.4	3.8
FIGS, DRIED	3 small (24 g)	62	0.9	15.9	0.3	2.4
GRAPEFRUIT	1 whole (246 g)	104	1.8	26.2	0.4	4.0
GRAPES, SEEDLESS	1 cup (151 g)	104	1.1	27.3	0.2	1.4
HONEYDEW	1 cup cubed (170 g)	61	0.9	56.1	0.2	1.4
KIWI	2 medium (152 g)	92	1.8	22.2	0.8	4.6
MANGO	1 whole (207 g)	135	1.1	35.2	0.6	3.7
NECTARINE	1 large (156 g)	69	1.7	16.5	0.5	2.7
ORANGE	1 large (184 g)	86	1.7	21.6	0.2	4.4
PAPAYA	1.5 cups, cubed (140 g)	83	1.3	20.5	0.3	3.7
PEACH	1 large (175 g)	68	1.6	17.3	0.4	2.6
PEAR	1 medium (178 g)	103	0.7	27.5	0.2	5.5
PINEAPPLE, FRESH	1 cup chunks (165 g)	82	0.9	21.6	0.2	2.3
PLUMS, FRESH	2 whole (132 g)	60	1.0	15	0.4	1.8
PRUNES (DRIED PLUMS)	3 whole (30 g)	69	0.6	18.3	0.6	2.1
RAISINS	¼ cup (43 g)	129	1.3	34.0	0.2	1.6
RASPBERRIES	1 cup (123 g)	64	1.5	14.7	0.8	8.0
STRAWBERRIES	1.5 cups, whole (216 g)	69	1.2	16.6	0.6	4.4
TANGERINES (MANDARIN ORANGES)	2 medium (176 g)	93	1.4	23.4	0.6	3.2
WATERMELON	1.5 cups, cubed (231 g)	68.4	1.2	17.3	0.3	1.0

CHAPTER 7

THE ONE WITH ALL
THE FINE PRINT

LAN AND I DON'T KNOW YOU. Not personally, that is. But if you belong to a gym, or spend much time online reading about training and nutrition, or have tried to gain or lose weight, we know a lot of people like you. So we can guess you already have questions for Alan in five general areas.

▶ Meal frequency

▶ Nutrient timing

▶ Supplements

▶ Alcohol

▶ The 10 percent of daily calories that fall into Alan's "pure junky goodness" category

We'll tackle them in that order.

Does Meal Frequency Matter?

Short answer? No, not really. At least, not in the way you think. But this is such a ripe area for mythology and countermythology, bunking and debunking, that it's worth taking a few minutes to look at what we actually do and don't know about meal frequency.

Alan and I entered the fitness industry about the same time, in the early 1990s. Back then there was a popular analogy: Your body's metabolism is a fire, and the more frequently you stoke it with fuel, the more consistently it will burn. You know that throwing a big log on a fire will temporarily tamp down the blaze, while a steady supply of kindling will keep it going just the way you like it: hot and steady.

It was a beautiful analogy; Alan repeated it to his personal-training clients, and my fellow editors and I used it in countless articles and books. You could identify a serious gym rat by the Tupperware meals he carried with him in a cooler. He knew, as we all knew back then, that if you didn't eat small, frequent meals, your metabolism would slow down.

The formula was based on tradition and social proof. It's what really lean bodybuilders and fitness models did, so it must work. But there was no evidence to back it up. When researchers experimented by isolating volunteers in metabolic chambers and measuring every calorie they took in or expended, they found no difference caused by the number of meals. It didn't matter if it was two, seven, or anything in between. If calories were kept constant, so was the metabolic rate.

One recent study compared 3 to 14 meals a day (yes, 14!) and found no difference in either fat or carbohydrate usage over 36 hours.

That said, some research has shown that an irregular number of meals—two on Monday, five on Tuesday, for example—will lead to metabolic consequences. You'll burn fewer calories after eating and tend to have reduced insulin sensitivity. Which raises an obvious follow-up question: Does this apply to all the people who practice intermittent fasting, going without food altogether for up to 24 hours at a time? That's probably a stretch. The ones we know who're into this type of fasting are all regular exercisers, which is known to improve insulin sensitivity and other health markers.

Meal Frequency and Protein Synthesis

The bodybuilders we knew back in the day, the ones who brought tuna and chicken breasts everywhere they went, were worried about more than their metabolic rate. Their goal was to create near-constant muscle-protein synthesis, with the idea that feeding muscles more frequently would make them grow more steadily. The most hard core, according to legend, would actually wake up in the middle of the night to eat. I can't say which they feared more:

their muscles missing an opportunity to grow, or an 8-hour fast causing them to shrink. (I also can't say if anybody actually did this; the stories I heard were told for comic relief, rather than instruction.)

Researchers who looked at it over a 12-hour period found the greatest protein synthesis occurred when young lifters ate 20 grams of protein four times in a day, with 3 hours between feedings. That worked better than eight 10-gram feedings or two with 40 grams.

This may be an example of the *leucine threshold,* a relatively new concept in exercise science. We touched on leucine, the most powerful amino acid, in Chapter 2, and in Chapter 6 we showed how much leucine you get from standard serving sizes of protein-rich foods. A meal with 20 to 30 grams of high-quality protein will typically offer 2 to 3 grams of leucine, which should switch on protein synthesis as high as it can go. The exception is older lifters (men in their seventies), who may need as much as 35 to 40 protein grams to get the full effect.

Meal Frequency and Body Composition

While acute, short-term studies don't support the idea that frequent meals "stoke the metabolic furnace" any better than eating less often, longer-term studies suggest it's still an open question. The best example is a 2013 study in *Obesity,* which showed that men who ate a high-protein diet (a third of total calories) spread over six daily meals lost more fat than a matched group eating three meals a day.

But What about Breakfast?

I'm a morning person and lifelong breakfast eater, so I never really questioned the primacy of breakfast as the most important meal of the day. An extensive body of research correlates breakfast eating with better weight control, while breakfast skipping is typically associated with every negative health outcome short of traumatic brain injury. But you know what they say about how correlation doesn't equal causation? The fact most healthy people in surveys claim to do something doesn't mean that particular behavior or practice is what makes them healthy.

So it goes with breakfast. When researchers experiment with calorie distribution throughout the day—front-loading or back-loading calories, eating or not eating breakfast, eating carbs earlier or later in the day—the results are all over the place. Alan looked at seven studies, published between 1987 and 2013, and found no pattern.

As we write this, in early 2014, there doesn't seem to be any cause-and-effect link between breakfast eating and weight control. Alan says the evidence isn't compelling enough for you to change lifelong habits and preferences. If you don't like eating breakfast, you can reach your goals without it. If you're more like me, and wake up hungry every morning, there's no problem with that either.

Nutrient Timing

The idea of an "anabolic window of opportunity" emerged in the late 1980s. Originally, research suggested that athletes needed to consume fast-acting carbs within 1 hour of a glycogen-depleting workout; otherwise they wouldn't completely recover their energy stores. We later learned this was an issue only for athletes who needed that glycogen later the same day. If you had 24 hours to replenish, it didn't really matter when you ate. By then a similar but more powerful idea had taken hold: If you don't eat protein soon after training, the anabolic window of opportunity closes.

A 2004 book called *Nutrient Timing: The Future of Sports Nutrition* cemented this idea among scientists, nutritionists, trainers, fitness writers, and, of course, serious gym rats worldwide. The authors wrote that the specific and precise timing of nutrients helps lifters "avoid the plateau effect and achieve far greater gains in muscle strength and muscle mass." Alan and I both have dog-eared and highlighted copies, and for years we didn't question its conclusions.

The conclusions weren't wrong; the research available at the time showed that timing mattered. Problem was, the conclusions were based on acute studies, often with subjects who hadn't eaten anything in the previous 12 hours. There was still an open question: Does protein synthesis in the first few hours after a workout accurately reflect how much muscles grow over weeks or months? More recent studies looked at the longer-term effects on lifters who were eating the way lifters generally do—that is, they were getting a lot of protein throughout the day and weren't typically training on an empty stomach.

Alan and Brad Schoenfeld tackled this topic in a review published in 2013 in the *Journal of the International Society of Sports Nutrition*. While acknowledging that timing matters, they argue that the "anabolic window" is quite a bit larger than most of us believed: 4 to 6 hours, counting the food you eat before training. That pre-workout food takes several hours to work its way through your system, which means it's still there immediately post-workout. Another meal within the next several hours should cover your needs.

Is the issue closed? No. As Alan explains, the research we have covers a limited range of possibilities: protein eaten within an hour pre- and/or post-training versus protein eaten 2 or more hours before or after. There could be a more powerful effect of timing that simply hasn't yet been studied.

Based on what we know today, it looks like total protein intake matters most. Which, of course, is what Alan has emphasized throughout this book. But to be clear, the question of timing has no single, black-and-white, one-size-fits-all answer. Alan sees its importance as a continuum.

MINIMAL IMPORTANCE	VARIABLE IMPORTANCE	MAXIMAL IMPORTANCE
Overweight/obese persons seeking weight loss for general health	Advanced/competitive trainees looking to push the limits of hypertrophy, strength, or fat loss	Competitions involving more than one glycogen-depleting event in a single day, separated by only a few hours
Novice and intermediate lifters seeking to improve body composition	Exhaustive/continuous training sessions that occur shortly after an overnight fast	Competitions or training bouts that significantly exceed 2 hours, especially bouts that approach or exceed 3 hours
Non-fasted resistance-training bouts lasting 1 hour or less	Exhaustive/continuous training sessions that significantly exceed 1 hour, especially sessions that approach 2 hours	
Noncompetitive training sessions or events		
Goals that do not involve endurance competition		
Goals that do not involve extremes in muscle gain or fat loss		

Supplements

Most of the studies on nutrient timing have involved protein supplements, with or without fast-acting carbohydrates. And we'll get to those in a moment. Let's start with something much simpler: multivitamins. They're probably the first supplement you took as a kid, and there's a decent chance you never stopped taking them. As Alan noted back in Chapter 2, if you're basically healthy and well nourished, a multivitamin is unlikely to make you healthier and *better* nourished.

But we also noted that people who aggressively cut calories—from bodybuilders to regular guys following a popular diet—probably are deficient in *something*. A few others who may need supplemental vitamins:

POPULATION	POTENTIALLY LACKING . . .
Obese and/or poor individuals, especially those who eat a lot of processed food	Multiple vitamins and minerals
People with dark-colored skin	Vitamin D
Those who cover skin or use sunscreen whenever outside	Vitamin D
Older adults	Vitamins B_{12} and D, zinc
Alcoholics	Vitamins A and B, various minerals
Smokers	Vitamins C and E
Vegans and others who limit animal foods	Vitamins B_{12} and D, calcium, iron, zinc
People who have no excuse for eating a crappy diet	Multiple vitamins and minerals

Fish Oil

A few years back, a friend sent me a link to one of the first mainstream articles that questioned the value of vitamins for otherwise healthy adults. While both of us marveled at the turnaround—if anything in nutrition science seemed safe from second-guessing, my money would have been on multivitamins—we wondered what was next. My guess was fish oil. At the time, fish oil was the LeBron James of supplements. It was linked to a lower risk of depression, better brain function, and healthier joints—and those were some of the *lesser* benefits, comparable to LeBron's ball-handling skills. The cardiovascular benefits were the big selling points: lower risk of inflammation, improved blood pressure, lower triglycerides, better overall blood-flow, and lower risk of heart attack and stroke. A 2011 study even suggested that fish oil builds muscle.

But in 2012, a meta-analysis of the available research came to an unexpected conclusion: Omega-3 fatty acids, usually consumed in the form of fish oil, didn't reduce the risk of heart failure, stroke, or death from any cause. That was immediately followed by another review, which came to the opposite conclusion: Fish oil reduced the risk of any type of cardiovascular event by 10 percent, and the overall risk of death by 5 percent. And then a more recent review, published in 2013, kind of split the difference, which is as close as scientists ever get to saying, "Yeah, sure. Why not?"

Your best move: As Alan said in Chapter 2, eat fatty fish at least three times a week, or take three to six fish-oil capsules a day.

Vitamin D

The argument for supplementing with vitamin D is strong.

- ▶ More than 40 percent of American adults are thought to be deficient.

- ▶ As more of us spend longer hours indoors and are more likely to wear sunscreen when we go out, we have less sun exposure, which is the strongest and most reliable source of vitamin D.

- ▶ Milk consumption in the United States has declined 30 percent since 1975, cutting off another traditional source.

Or, I should say, it would be strong if we could link supplemental D to positive health outcomes. New research casts doubt, showing it doesn't prevent osteoporosis—long assumed to be a potential consequence of declining milk consumption—or other diseases, like colorectal cancer. The chicken-and-egg question remains open: Are the diseases linked to low levels of vitamin D caused by that deficiency? Or is the deficiency caused by the same mechanisms that create the disease?

On the other hand, some recent research suggests D supplements help muscles recover from training, and may also increase testosterone.

Alan recommends supplementing with 3,000 to 4,000 IU a day for those hormonal benefits, or 1,000 to 2,000 IU a day if you're worried about a deficiency.

Magnesium

How well your body uses vitamin D is tied to your magnesium intake. And that's just one of 300-plus metabolic processes in which magnesium plays a part. Low levels are linked to a long list of diseases, including type 2 diabetes. Magnesium, like D, is chronically underconsumed by more than 40 percent of Americans. Basic multivitamins aren't much help; as we noted in Chapter 2, they typically aren't big enough to include the full 400 milligrams recommended for adult men. If you don't want to supplement, nuts and seeds are among the best food sources, along with tubers, whole grains, and dark, leafy greens.

Supplementing for Size and Strength

It's a lot easier to talk about supplements for increasing size than for decreasing it. That's because there's not a lot of evidence to believe any fat-burning supplement offers real benefits beyond what you'll get from your diet and workouts. The most effective ones, like ephedra and caffeine, fall on the wrong side of the risk-reward equation.

So let's talk about the ones associated with muscle hypertrophy and strength. Here's a summary from the International Society of Sports Nutrition.

STRENGTH OF EVIDENCE	MUSCLE-BUILDING	PERFORMANCE-ENHANCING
Apparently effective and generally safe	Creatine Protein Essential amino acids (EAA) Weight gain powders	Creatine Carbohydrates Caffeine Beta-alanine Sodium bicarbonate Water and sports drinks Sodium phosphate

STRENGTH OF EVIDENCE	MUSCLE-BUILDING	PERFORMANCE-ENHANCING
Possibly effective	HMB (a metabolite of leucine) Branched-chain amino acids (BCAA)	Post-exercise carbohydrates and protein EAA BCAA HMB Glycerol
Too early to tell	α-ketoglutarate α-ketoisocaproate Ecdysterones Growth hormone–releasing peptides and secretagogues Ornithine α-ketoglutarate Zinc/magnesium aspartate	Medium-chain triglycerides
Apparently dangerous and/or not effective	Glutamine Smilax Isoflavones Sulfo-polysaccharides (myostatin inhibitors) Boron Chromium Conjugated linoleic acid Gamma oryzanol Prohormones Tribulus terrestris Vanadyl sulfate (vanadium)	Glutamine Ribose Inosine

Don't worry if two-thirds of the chart reads like that chemistry test you forgot to study for. (And if you're waiting for those nightmares about college exams to go away, I'm here to tell you they don't: I still have them more than 20 years post–grad school.) You can go the rest of your life without knowing anything more about inosine and vanadyl sulfate than you do now. The important information is at the top.

It shows that your best bets are creatine and protein. Especially protein, since it includes EAA (essential amino acids), BCAA (branched-chain amino acids), weight gain powders, and post-exercise protein and carbohydrates. Your protein shakes may or may not include much carbohydrate (especially in the massive quantities you'll find in weight gain powders), but they certainly have enough of the key amino acids to maximize protein synthesis.

But you already know that, since we've mentioned protein so many times you probably wonder if we're getting paid to endorse it. (We aren't, beyond some free products here and there—which, for the record, we really appreciate.) This chart shows why whey protein powder is such an effective tool for a guy who wants more muscle than he has now.

PROTEIN QUALITY RANKINGS

PROTEIN TYPE	PROTEIN EFFICIENCY RATIO	BIOLOGICAL VALUE	NET PROTEIN UTILIZATION	PROTEIN DIGESTIBILITY CORRECTED AMINO ACID SCORE
BEEF	2.9	80	73	0.92
BLACK BEANS	0	(no data)	0	0.75
CASEIN	2.5	77	76	1.00
EGG	3.9	100	94	1.00
MILK	2.5	91	82	1.00
PEANUTS	1.8	(no data)	(no data)	0.52
SOY PROTEIN	2.2	74	61	1.00
WHEAT GLUTEN	0.8	64	67	0.25
WHEY PROTEIN	3.2	104	92	1.00

The four protein-rating systems each measure something slightly different, but all come to the same basic conclusions about which proteins are easiest for your body to digest and use. (The higher the number, the better.) You see the highest scores for eggs and whey. When you don't have time to cook, you can't really go wrong with a basic whey protein supplement from an established company.

Now, about creatine . . .

You probably know it occurs naturally in your body, with 95 percent of it stored in your muscles. It provides energy for high-intensity, short-duration activities. We get some from meat and seafood, but creatine supplements, which have been around since the early 1990s, give us an easy and safe way to increase our natural stores. The extra creatine helps you get an additional rep or two on your heaviest sets, and most lifters find their strength increases about 10 percent with supplementation. Muscle mass should increase by about 4 pounds over several months of consistent use.

Basic creatine monohydrate supplements are the least expensive and most reliable. In the early days it was assumed you needed to "load" with 20 grams of creatine a day for a week, and that it wouldn't work without heavy infusions of sugar. Now we know you can saturate your muscles with 2 to 3 grams a day for 30 days. There's no known benefit to taking more than your muscles can hold.

Alcohol

Here's an evolutionary factoid that should blow your mind: Humans, as noted in Chapter 4, separated from chimpanzees at least 5 million years ago. Both species have some ability to metabolize alcohol. Scientists have observed drunken primates in the wild, a consequence of eating overripe, naturally fermented fruit, which has an alcohol content similar to beer. And, of course, all of us have observed drunken primates of the domesticated variety, a consequence of drinking just about anything with a surgeon general's warning on the label. But here's the mind-blowing part: Research suggests that the genes to metabolize alcohol go back 10 million years, to an ancestor that may predate both chimps and humans.

Which is why popular culture's least evolved male, Homer Simpson, was able to sum up our feelings so eloquently: "To alcohol! The cause of, and solution to, all of life's problems."

Now, if alcohol is *literally* the cause of any of your problems, past or present, the best advice is to avoid it entirely. And if you haven't started to drink it, no one recommends that you should. But since 100 percent of this book's authors enjoy the occasional cold one, we feel comfortable pointing out that moderate alcohol consumption is linked to a long list of health benefits. We'll leave it to others to decide if those health benefits come from the alcohol itself or the fact that moderate drinkers tend to do lots of things moderately, and are more likely to have the education and socioeconomic status linked to good health.

Moderate drinking is unlikely to affect your weight in either direction, as long as the calories in alcohol replace something else. If they don't, you'll probably gain fat. Here's the damage.

SERVING SIZE AND TYPE	CALORIES (KCAL)	GRAMS OF ALCOHOL
12-OZ BEER	153	13.9
12-OZ LIGHT BEER	103	11
5-OZ WINE (RED)	125	15.6
5-OZ WINE (WHITE)	121	15.1
3-OZ SAKE	117	14.1
1.5-OZ HARD LIQUOR (80 PROOF, OR 40% ALCOHOL)	97	14

Alan suggests swapping out carbs for alcohol. So if you drink two beers, that's 300 calories, and about 75 carbohydrate grams. The swap works best if you choose a higher percentage of carbs in your meal plan. If you've chosen lower carbs, you may have to take away from your fat allotment. That's a worse choice, Alan says, because dietary fat is essential for functions that contribute to a better physique, like testosterone production.

Beer drinkers, thus, may be tempted to switch to wine, which has more alcohol per serving with fewer calories. But keep in mind that 5 ounces is a minuscule pour, and looks even punier in the glassware many bars and restaurants now use. If it takes three of them to replace two beers, you have to find even more calories to cut.

Crap

You know by now that 10 percent of your diet can come from anything that's legal to consume. To qualify for Alan's "pure junky goodness" rubric, it has to be far removed from its natural state, no matter if it's been processed for flavor, or to remain edible following a nuclear conflagration, or some combination. Those calories have to come from somewhere, and once again Alan suggests you start with your carbohydrate allotment, rather than fat. (Protein is pretty much nonnegotiable.)

Let's say your junk allotment comes to 250 calories—10 percent of your daily total of 2,500. You already know that's not even two beers' worth. It's one Snickers bar. A serving of ice cream is 150 calories, which sounds promising only until you realize the serving size is one-half cup. Double that and it still doesn't seem like a real dessert (to me, anyway), but even that dainty little dollop takes you over the daily allotment.

You have the option of banking those calories and using several days' worth on a treat that actually seems like a treat. So let's say you save up 3 days' worth. Those 750 calories get you a slice of New York cheesecake at Ruby Tuesday.

That brings us to a bombshell revelation, which we saved for the end of the chapter to reward those who are still reading: Alan doesn't *really* expect you to stick with the 10 percent limitation on junk food. Not all the time, anyway.

It's great if you can, but it's more aspirational than operational. As we've asserted so many times already, the keys to the Lean Muscle Plan are, in this order.

1. Hitting your target for total calories

2. Hitting your macronutrient targets, especially for protein

3. Getting almost all your food from whole and minimally processed sources

Get those three right, and a little more junk won't necessarily show up in your trunk.

CHAPTER 8:

THE ONE WITH ALL THE SAMPLE MEAL PLANS

THESE MEAL PLANS won't look like any you've seen before, unless you've seen one of Alan's in your travels. Alan prides himself on packing as much information as he can into the smallest possible space, giving you the ability to take in the entire plan at a single glance. We obviously haven't skimped on any details; that's why you bought the book. But we also wanted to make sure the plan fits on pages you can photocopy or print from your home computer. You can highlight it, bring it with you on business trips and vacations, memorize it, frame it for posterity.

You'll immediately notice that the main meals are listed as A, B, and C, rather than breakfast, lunch, and dinner. They're all "floating" meals; you can eat them in any order that works for you. Same with the snacks—they can be eaten at any time, in any order, or in any combination. If you prefer to eat less often, just add food from the snacks to your main meals.

A Quick Note about Fats

In the main meals, Alan assumes a small amount of fat will go into the meal, in the form of cooking oil, salad dressing, or some other condiment or flavoring. If you don't use any additional fat, your meals will be a bit lighter than the plan calls for. In Alan's experience, that's never been a problem, even for clients who were trying to gain weight.

He also doesn't account for fish-oil supplements, since some of you don't need or want to take them. Yes, three to six capsules a day is an extra 3 to 6 grams of fat, which is 27 to 54 calories, but again it's never been an issue for Alan's clients.

Fluid

Most of us drink far more than we need, which, if nothing else, gives us peace of mind in knowing our toilets are in good working order. You don't have to go out of your way to drink when you aren't thirsty. A good target is 16 to 32 ounces of noncaloric fluid a day, in addition to whatever you drink during or after exercise. Coffee, tea, and diet sodas count toward that total. (Although I'm a heavy consumer of Coke Zero, Alan is not a fan.)

Variety: Alan's Rule of Two

Try to eat at least two different foods within each of Alan's six food groups.

<u>Meg</u>'s = Meat and other protein-rich foods

<u>Fa</u>bulous = Fat-rich foods

<u>Fi</u>gure = Fibrous vegetables

<u>St</u>opped = Starchy foods

<u>Mi</u>ssing = Milk and other dairy products

<u>Fr</u>ies = Fruits

It's really more of a guideline than a rule, and probably matters more for the fruits and vegetables than any other category. A mix of colors—oranges and kiwis, broccoli and bell peppers—guarantees a wider range of vitamins and minerals.

Timing Meals around Workouts

The easiest strategy is to have the workout fall between two of your main meals. So you'd eat one meal within 2 hours of training, and the next within

2 hours postworkout. That ensures your muscles have plenty of protein available when they need it.

Guys who work out first thing in the morning have a trickier decision. If your primary goal is fat loss, there shouldn't be a problem with training on an empty stomach, as long as you eat a main meal soon after. If you're trying to gain weight, Alan recommends eating at least a little protein before, or protein with carbs if the workout includes some endurance work. Then have a main meal within 2 hours of training.

Measuring vs. Ballparking

Life is imprecise. When you have to eat on the run, or have lunch with co-workers, or enjoy a night out with family or friends, the meals won't fit the *Lean Muscle Diet* templates. The key to success is to control what you can, when you can. If a restaurant meal differs significantly from your plan, try to make up for it later.

When you're at home, or planning meals and snacks for work, it's important to get objective measurements of how much you're eating. Break out the measuring cups and spoons, at least for the first 2 to 3 weeks. By then you should be able to judge serving sizes and proportions with a glance.

You don't have to worry about weighing meat on a scale. For meat and fish, your hand is good enough. (Just like . . . you know.) A slab the size and thickness of your palm will be about 6 ounces. If it's the size and thickness of your four fingers, it's about 3 ounces. Adjust accordingly if your hands are unusually large or small.

Ultimately, Alan says, consistency matters most. Even if you mismeasure your portions, or fail to measure them at all, you want to do it consistently. That is, make sure your portions look to be about the same size and feel equally light or heavy, both on your plate and in your stomach. Note how long it takes between meals to get hungry again. Those are all data points. Even if they aren't *accurate* data points, you have a basis to judge your results as long as their inaccuracy stays in the same ballpark.

Not losing fat or gaining muscle as fast as you think you should? Okay, now it's time to measure more carefully, and make sure you're really on *the* plan, and not just *a* plan.

How to Fit In Your Indulgences

To Alan, this is both an art and a science: "It must—I repeat, *must!*—be dictated by personal preference." But that doesn't mean there aren't better and worse ways to do it. Your best strategy: A cup of cooked starchy food—beans, rice, pasta—will be right around 200 calories. That's the first place to make a swap. Alan will show specific examples for each of the four case studies on the following pages.

CASE STUDY #1: DESKBOUND DAN

Current status: 240 pounds, novice lifter, sedentary

Goal: Lose 24 pounds in 6 months

Daily targets:

▶ 2,592 calories

▶ 216 grams of protein

▶ 139 grams of carbs

▶ 130 grams of fat

FLOATING MEAL A: 425 calories, 25 g protein, 25 g carbs, 25 g fat

▶ Three whole eggs, cooked any style (or) 3 ounces moderate- or high-fat meat, any type (or) 3 ounces very lean meat + $1/4$ cup nuts, any type (or) 1 scoop protein powder + 2 tablespoons nut butter, any type (or) 1 scoop protein powder + $1/4$ cup nuts, any type (or) 1 cup low-fat cottage cheese + 1 tablespoon nut butter, any type

▶ 1 serving of fruit: one large fruit, any type, such as apple, banana, or orange (or) $1^1/2$ cups fresh fruit (or) $1/3$ cup dried fruit (or) two small fruits, such as apricots, figs, tangerines, or kiwis

▶ Fibrous veggies can be added if/as desired; shoot for at least 3 servings total for the day (a serving of fibrous veggies is approximately 1 cup).

FLOATING MEAL B: 544 calories, 48 g protein, 43 g carbs, 20 g fat

- ▶ 6 ounces very lean to moderate-fat meat (or) 2 scoops protein powder + $1/_8$ cup nuts (a scant handful), any type (or) 2 cups tofu, firm (or) 2 scoops protein powder + 1 tablespoon nut butter, any type

- ▶ 1 cup cooked measurement of any starch, such as rice, pasta, peas, beans, corn, oatmeal, or grits (or) 1 cup ready-to-eat dry cereal, any type (or) two slices of bread, any type (or) one mid-size potato, any type, roughly 6 to 7 ounces

- ▶ Fibrous veggies can be added if/as desired; shoot for at least 3 servings total for the day (a serving of fibrous veggies is approximately 1 cup).

FLOATING SNACKS: 924 calories, 57 g protein, 48 g carbs, 56 g fat

- ▶ 4 ounces very lean meat (or) $1^{1}/_2$ scoops protein powder

- ▶ $2/_3$ cup nuts, any type (or) 4 tablespoons nut butter, any type

- ▶ 1 serving of full-fat cheese, any type (a serving is one slice, $1/_8$ cup, or a 1-inch cube). Note: Any dairy serving (1 cup milk, $3/_4$ cup yogurt, or 1 ounces cheese) will do here; cheese just happens to fit closer to the macro target. Minor deviations are inconsequential.

- ▶ 1 serving of fruit: one large fruit, any type, such as apple, banana, or orange (or) $1^{1}/_2$ cups fresh fruit (or) $1/_3$ cup dried fruit (or) two small fruits, such as apricots, figs, tangerines, or kiwis

FLOATING MEAL C: 702 calories, 86 g protein, 22 g carbs, 30 g fat

- ▶ 12 ounces very lean to moderate-fat meat

- ▶ $1/_2$ cup cooked measurement of any starch, such as rice, pasta, peas, beans, corn, or oatmeal (or) $1/_2$ cup dry cereal, any type (or) one slice of bread, any type (or) half a midsize potato, any type (or) one small potato, any type, roughly 3 ounces

- ▶ Fibrous veggies can be added if/as desired; shoot for at least 3 servings total for the day (a serving of fibrous veggies is approximately 1 cup).

How Dan Gets His Junk On

Dan can use up to 10 percent of his daily calories for any earthly pleasure that's loosely defined as "edible" and has calories that can be measured. ***Best choice:*** In Meal B he has 1 cup of starch, which is roughly 200 calories, or 8 percent of his total. That buys him 5 Twizzlers. ***Second-best choice:*** He can take the starch from meals B and C; that's $1^1/_2$ cups of cereal or pasta, or three slices of bread. It's about 300 calories, 12 percent of his total, which is 1 cup of ice cream.

CASE STUDY #2: SKINNY-FAT STAN

Current status: 160 pounds, novice lifter, somewhat active

Goal: Simultaneously shed 12 pounds of fat and gain 12 pounds of muscle in 6 months

Daily targets:

▶ 2,560 calories

▶ 160 grams of protein

▶ 264 grams of carbs

▶ 96 grams of fat

FLOATING MEAL A: 425 calories, 25 g protein, 25 g carbs, 25 g fat

▶ Three whole eggs, cooked any style (or) 3 ounces moderate or high-fat meat, any type (or) 3 ounces very lean meat + $^1/_4$ cup nuts, any type (or) 1 scoop protein powder + 2 tablespoons nut butter, any type (or) 1 scoop protein powder + $^1/_4$ cup nuts, any type (or) 1 cup low-fat cottage cheese + 1 tablespoon nut butter, any type

▶ 1 serving of fruit: one large fruit, any type, such as apple, banana, or orange (or) $1^1/_2$ cups fresh fruit (or) $^1/_3$ cup dried fruit (or) two small fruits, such as apricots, figs, tangerines, or kiwis

▶ Fibrous veggies can be added if/as desired; shoot for at least 3 servings total for the day (a serving of fibrous veggies is approximately 1 cup).

FLOATING MEAL B: 689 calories, 38 g protein, 87 g carbs, 21 g fat

▶ 4 ounces very lean to moderate-fat meat (or) 1½ cups tofu, firm (or) 1½ scoops protein powder + ⅛ cup nuts (a scant handful), any type (or) 1½ scoops protein powder + 1 tablespoon nut butter, any type (or) 1 cup low-fat cottage cheese

▶ 2 cups cooked measurement of any starch, such as rice, pasta, peas, beans, corn, oatmeal, or grits (or) 2 cups dry cereal, any type (or) 2 midsize potatoes, 6 to 7 ounces each, any type (or) 4 small potatoes, 3 ounces each, any type

▶ Fibrous veggies can be added if/as desired; shoot for at least 3 servings total for the day (a serving of fibrous veggies is approximately 1 cup).

FLOATING SNACKS: 684 calories, 48 g protein, 60 g carbs, 28 g fat

▶ 3 ounces very lean meat (or) 1 scoop protein powder (or) 1 cup fat-free Greek yogurt

▶ ⅓ cup nuts, any type (or) 3 tablespoons nut butter, any type

▶ 2 servings low-fat milk and/or yogurt (1 serving = 1 cup milk or ¾ cup yogurt). Note: Any dairy will do here; milk and yogurt just happen to fit closer to the macro target. Minor deviations are inconsequential.

▶ 1 serving of fruit: one large fruit, any type, such as apple, banana, or orange (or) 1½ cups fresh fruit (or) ⅓ cup dried fruit (or) two small fruits, such as apricots, figs, tangerines, or kiwis

FLOATING MEAL C: 759 calories, 50 g protein, 88 g carbs, 23 g fat

▶ 6 ounces very lean to moderate-fat meat (or) 2 cups tofu, firm (or) 2 scoops protein powder + ⅛ cup nuts (a scant handful), any type (or) 2 scoops protein powder + 1 tablespoon nut butter, any type

▶ 2 cups cooked measurement of any starch, such as rice, pasta, peas, beans, corn, oatmeal, or grits (or) 2 cups dry cereal, any type (or) two midsize potatoes, 6 to 7 ounces each, any type (or) four small potatoes, 3 ounces each, any type

▶ Fibrous veggies can be added if/as desired; shoot for at least 3 servings total for the day (a serving of fibrous veggies is approximately 1 cup).

How Stan Gets His Junk On

Similar to Dan, Stan has about 250 calories a day to play with. Unlike Dan, he has a lot of starchy carbs to swap out. But let's imagine Stan as a bit of a hedonist. If he takes 1 cup of starch from meals B and C, he has 400 calories, which is just over 15 percent of his total. That gets him a slice of reduced-fat banana–chocolate chip coffee cake at Starbucks.

CASE STUDY #3: BROTACULAR BOB

Current status: 190 pounds, experienced lifter, active

Goal: Lose 10 pounds of fat in 6 months without sacrificing any strength or size

Daily targets:

▶ 2,610 calories

▶ 180 grams of protein

▶ 270 grams of carbs

▶ 90 grams of fat

FLOATING MEAL A: 380 calories, 25 g protein, 25 g carbs, 20 g fat

▶ Three whole eggs, cooked any style (or) 3 ounces very lean to moderate-fat meat, any type (or) 3 ounces very lean meat + $\frac{1}{4}$ cup nuts, any type (or) 1 scoop protein powder + 2 tablespoons nut butter, any type (or) 1 scoop protein powder + $\frac{1}{4}$ cup nuts, any type (or) 1 cup low-fat cottage cheese + 1 tablespoon nut butter, any type

- ▶ 1 serving of fruit: one large fruit, any type, such as apple, banana, pear, or orange (or) $1^1/_2$ cups fresh fruit (or) $^1/_3$ cup dried fruit (or) two small fruits, such as apricots, figs, dates, plums, tangerines, or kiwis

- ▶ Fibrous veggies can be added if/as desired; shoot for at least 3 servings total for the day (a serving of fibrous veggies is approximately 1 cup).

FLOATING MEAL B: 759 calories, 50 g protein, 88 g carbs, 23 g fat

- ▶ 6 ounces very lean to moderate-fat meat (or) 2 cups tofu, firm (or) 2 scoops protein powder + $^1/_8$ cup nuts (a scant handful), any type (or) 2 scoops protein powder + 1 tablespoon nut butter, any type

- ▶ 2 cups cooked measurement of any starch, such as rice, pasta, peas, beans, corn, oatmeal, or grits (or) 2 cups dry cereal, any type (or) two mid-size potatoes, 6 to 7 ounces each, any type (or) four small potatoes, 3 ounces each, any type

- ▶ Fibrous veggies can be added if/as desired; shoot for at least 3 servings total for the day (a serving of fibrous veggies is approximately 1 cup).

FLOATING SNACKS: 693 calories, 56 g protein, 56 g carbs, 21 g fat

- ▶ 4 ounces very lean meat (or) $1^1/_2$ scoops protein powder (or) 1 cup low-fat cottage cheese

- ▶ 1 ounces nuts (slightly less than $^1/_4$ cup), any type (or) 2 tablespoon nut butter, any type

- ▶ 2 servings low-fat milk and/or yogurt (1 serving = 1 cup milk or $^3/_4$ cup yogurt). Note: Any dairy will do here; milk and yogurt just happen to fit closer to the macro target. Minor deviations are inconsequential.

- ▶ 1 serving of fruit: one large fruit, any type, such as apple, banana, or orange (or) $1^1/_2$ cups fresh fruit (or) $^1/_3$ cup dried fruit (or) two small fruits, such as apricots, figs, tangerines, or kiwis

FLOATING MEAL C: 759 calories, 52 g protein, 104 g carbs, 24 g fat

▶ 6 ounces very lean to moderate-fat meat (or) 2 cups tofu, firm (or) 2 scoops protein powder + $^1/_8$ cup nuts (a scant handful), any type (or) 2 scoops protein powder + 1 tablespoon nut butter, any type

▶ 2$^1/_2$ cups cooked measurement of any starch, such as rice, pasta, peas, beans, corn, oatmeal, or grits (or) 2$^1/_2$ cups dry cereal, any type (or) two and one half midsize potatoes, 6 to 7 ounces each, any type (or) five small potatoes, 3 ounces each, any type

▶ Fibrous veggies can be added if/as desired; shoot for at least 3 servings total for the day (a serving of fibrous veggies is approximately 1 cup).

How Bob Gets His Junk On

You've probably noticed a theme here: Our first three case studies all end up with calorie allotments in the 2,500 to 2,600 range. But you see big differences in their macronutrients—from 216 grams of protein for Deskbound Dan to 160 grams for Skinny-Fat Stan. And while Dan has just 139 grams of carbs per day, Bob here has twice as many.

Bob, as it happens, is a social animal. On weekends he loves nothing more than surfing with his buds in the morning and then watching a game that afternoon. But he hates having to reveal he's on a diet. So Bob is going to save up all 1,820 calories for that one perfect day each week. Here's what he can get.

▶ An order of fire-grilled corn guacamole and chips (1,180 calories) at Chili's, and four bottles of Sam Adams Boston Lager (640 calories) = 1,820 calories

▶ Three slices of pizza (900 calories) + four mugs of Bud Light on tap (450 calories) + cake and ice cream at his nephew's birthday party that evening (470 calories) = 1,820 calories (okay, the birthday cake is a wild-ass guess)

▶ An order of baby back ribs (1,050 calories) with a side of sweet potato fries (450 calories) at Outback Steakhouse + two bottles of Flying Dog Doggie Style pale ale (320 calories) = 1,820 calories

CASE STUDY #4: BULKING BARRY

Current status: 160 pounds, extremely lean, incredibly active

Goal: Gain 10 pounds of solid muscle in 6 months without any fat

Daily targets:

▶ 3,230 calories

▶ 170 grams of protein

▶ 408 grams of carbs

▶ 102 grams of fat

FLOATING MEAL A: 683 calories, 34 g protein, 85 g carbs, 23 g fat

▶ Three whole eggs, cooked any style (or) 3 ounces very lean to moderate-fat meat, any type (or) 3 ounces very lean meat + ¼ cup nuts, any type (or) 1 scoop protein powder + 2 tablespoons nut butter, any type (or) 1 scoop protein powder + ¼ cup nuts, any type (or) 1 cup low-fat cottage cheese + 1 tablespoon nut butter, any type

▶ 2 cups cooked measurement of any starch, such as rice, pasta, peas, beans, corn, oatmeal, or grits (or) 1 cup ready-to-eat dry cereal, any type (or) two slices of bread, any type (or) one mid size potato, any type, roughly 6 to 7 ounces

▶ 1 serving of fruit: one large fruit, any type, such as apple, banana, or orange (or) 1½ cups fresh fruit (or) ⅓ cup dried fruit (or) two small fruits, such as apricots, figs, tangerines, or kiwis

▶ Fibrous veggies can be added if/as desired; shoot for at least 3 servings total for the day (a serving of fibrous veggies is approximately 1 cup).

FLOATING MEAL B: 689 calories, 38 g protein, 87 g carbs, 21 g fat

▶ 4 ounces very lean to moderate-fat meat (or) 1½ cups tofu, firm (or) 1½ scoops protein powder + ⅛ cup nuts (a scant handful), any type (or) 1½ scoops protein powder + 1 tablespoon nut butter, any type (or) 1 cup low-fat cottage cheese

▶ 2 cups cooked measurement of any starch, such as rice, pasta, peas, beans, corn, oatmeal, or grits (or) 2 cups dry cereal, any type (or) two mid size potatoes, 6 to 7 ounces each, any type (or) four small potatoes, 3 ounces each, any type

▶ Fibrous veggies can be added if/as desired; shoot for at least 3 servings total for the day (a serving of fibrous veggies is approximately 1 cup).

FLOATING SNACKS: 1,120 calories, 46 g protein, 117 g carbs, 32 g fat

▶ 2 cups cooked measurement of any starch, such as rice, pasta, peas, beans, corn, oatmeal, or grits (or) 2 cups dry cereal, any type (or) two mid size potatoes, 6 to 7 ounces each, any type (or) four small potatoes, 3 ounces each, any type

▶ ¼ cup nuts, any type (or) 2 tablespoon nut butter, any type

▶ 2 servings low-fat milk and/or yogurt (1 dairy serving = 1 cup milk or ¾ cup yogurt or 1 ounces cheese). Note: Any dairy will do here; milk and yogurt just happen to fit closer to the macro target. Minor deviations are inconsequential.

▶ 2 servings of fruit (1 serving = one large fruit), any type, such as apple, banana, or orange (or) 1½ cups fresh fruit (or) ⅓ cup dried fruit (or) two small fruits, such as apricots, figs, tangerines, or kiwis

FLOATING MEAL C: 921 calories, 54 g protein, 120 g carbs, 25 g fat

▶ 6 ounces very lean to moderate-fat meat (or) 2 cups tofu, firm (or) 2 scoops protein powder + ⅛ cup nuts (a scant handful), any type (or) 2 scoops protein powder + 1 tablespoon nut butter, any type

▶ 3 cups cooked measurement of any starch, such as rice, pasta, peas, beans, corn, oatmeal, or grits (or) 3 cups dry cereal, any type (or) three mid size potatoes, 6 to 7 ounces each, any type (or) six small potatoes, 3 ounces each, any type

▶ Fibrous veggies can be added if/as desired; shoot for at least 3 servings total for the day (a serving of fibrous veggies is approximately 1 cup).

How Barry Gets His Junk On

Remember back in Chapter 5, how we said Barry scares most people? As you can imagine, that puts a crimp in his social life. And since he doesn't have much of a sweet tooth, he doesn't see the point of cheat meals. A big indulgence for him is a pat of butter on his baked potato—not exactly a risky move, since his goal is to gain weight.

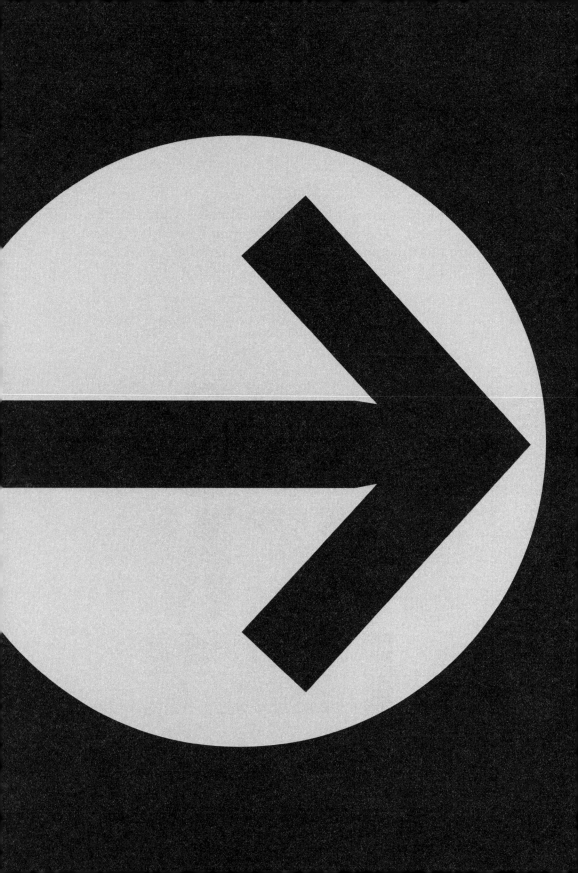

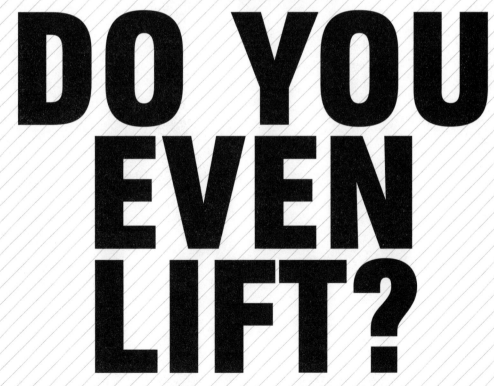

PART THREE:

DO YOU EVEN EVEN LIFT?

CHAPTER 9

HOW TO TRAIN

BEFORE WE CAN TALK ABOUT TRAINING, we need to define it. We often use it casually as a synonym for "working out" or, more generally, "exercise." I think we need to get more specific.

To me, *exercise* is movement you do for a reason. Maybe you take a walk on a Saturday afternoon because you feel like moving instead of sitting. Or you knock out some pushups during commercials while you watch a football game. Or you go to the driving range to hit a bucket, or shoot free throws in your driveway, or practice *kata* or sun salutations in your living room. That's exercise.

A *workout* is exercise you do to achieve a specific effect. You're trying to get your heart rate up, work up a sweat, burn calories, pump up the guns. Like generic exercise, a workout can be any length and involve any level of exertion, in service to any outcome you have in mind.

Training is a series of workouts you do to reach a goal, to achieve something you don't currently have. You're trying to get stronger than you are now, or bigger, or leaner, or faster. Most important, *you're taking planned, incremental steps toward that goal*. You're still getting exercise. You're still getting a good workout each time you go into the weight room. But you're doing it within the context of the plans you've made to reach a specific goal. Some days that means pushing yourself harder than you want to; other times it means pulling back a little: *not* hitting a personal best, *not* working yourself into a sweaty mess, *not* pumping your biceps until it feels like the skin on your arms is two sizes too small.

A training program can be simple or complex. The Lean Muscle Plan's is somewhere in between. But no program, no matter how sophisticated, will work unless you follow these basic laws of lifting.

1. Know exactly what you're going to do in your primary exercises before you start.

2. Remember that anything worth doing is worth warming up for.

3. Whatever matters most is what you do first.

4. Spend 80 percent of your time and energy on the exercises that matter most.

5. On each exercise, work with the heaviest weights you can within the context of the program.

This final point requires some clarification.

▶ Heavy means heavy for you. It's relative to your current strength and conditioning levels, and it's relative to when you do the exercise within the workout.

▶ If it's smaller than your forearm or lighter than your mother's purse, it's not heavy.

How the Program Works

You'll do three total-body workouts a week—the classic Monday-Wednesday-Friday or Tuesday-Thursday-Saturday schedule. You can do anything you want on the nonlifting days (more on that in a moment), as long as it doesn't involve heavy lifting. The three workouts have the same configuration but slightly different emphases.

Workouts 1 and 2 are your heavy workouts. Sometimes Workout 2 will have more of a hypertrophy emphasis, but you'll still push yourself to use heavier weights from week to week. Make sure you bring your testicles for these sessions, because you'll need them.

Workout 3 requires lighter weights (with a couple of exceptions, which you'll see in Chapter 11), but you'll generally do the exercises faster. Bring an absorbent gym towel, because you'll sweat buckets.

There are three phases to the program. How long a phase lasts will depend on how productive it is for you. Most readers will spend at least 4 weeks on each one. You want to keep going as long as you:

▶ Get stronger from week to week on one or more primary exercises

▶ Improve your form or endurance, or something else that matters to you

When you peak, and one week's workouts are no better than the previous week's, move on to the next phase. More advanced lifters may hit that wall in just 3 weeks. But entry-level readers might keep improving for months. Just remember that the goal of training is to make adaptations, and a workout is only as good as the adaptations it produces, while it's producing them.

Workout Structure

The workouts have three components.

1. Warmup. The most literal goal of a warmup routine is to raise your body's temperature by a couple degrees. Warmer muscles are less vulnerable to tears, and warm joints move better and with less friction.

More interesting is one of the least-known benefits of warming up: As you start to move, and your heart rate increases, so does your overall level of excitation. That's because your body is pumping out higher levels of hormones called catecholamines. They're associated with the fight-or-flight response to imminent danger, which is why we usually think of them as stress hormones. They're useful when we're on deadline, or being stalked by someone in a dark parking lot. We don't want to use too much of this system or use it too often, because in large doses it can suppress the immune system and leave us vulnerable to illness.

Training is a different kind of stress, one you impose on yourself to create adaptations that over time make you more resilient. That's where one of the catecholamines, adrenaline, is your secret weapon. Adrenaline makes you sharper and more focused. It releases some of the glycogen your liver has stored away for emergencies and opens up your blood vessels to get that extra fuel into your muscles. But it also releases subcutaneous fat, the kind you store between your muscles and skin. The stuff that jiggles. Now, you're not going to burn much fat during your warmup—in fact, it's the last thing you want to focus on—but you do want to start the process that enables it.

In addition to warming your body and activating those key hormones, a good warmup should also:

▶ Prepare your joints for the movements you'll use in the workout

▶ Activate your muscles

You'll see how to accomplish both in Chapter 10.

2. Core exercises. John Wooden, the legendary UCLA basketball coach, had a great quote: "The main ingredient of stardom is the rest of the team." When you train, the rest of the team includes your body's weakest links. The quirks of human physiology guarantee the lower torso is one of them.

Kevin McGinley, a reader of my books and articles, gave me a great layman's explanation of why we need to train for core stability: "If a structural engineer were to look at a human skeleton, he'd point to the gap between the hips and rib cage and say, 'That's your problem, right there.'"

It's not that your midsection isn't *potentially* strong; the best powerlifters can squat and deadlift three times their body weight. It's that there's so little margin for error. As I explained in Chapter 3, safety depends on stability, which means locking the lower back and pelvis into a neutral position, with the spine in its natural arch.

Most of us, left on our own, will do our core training at the end of the workout. If we do it last, it means we assign to it the least importance. I think it makes more sense to do those exercises early, right after the warmup but before the first heavy lifts of the day.

I see two benefits. The obvious one is that if you do these exercises first, you'll have more energy, and perform them better than you would at the end. Doing core exercises before heavy lifts also, I think, activates key stabilizing muscles without exhausting them to the point that they can't do their job when you need them most.

3. Strength exercises. This part of the workout includes six exercises, organized in two groups of three. The first group of three includes your primary exercises. In Workouts 1 and 2 you'll typically start with a deadlift or squat, followed by a push (pushup, bench press, shoulder press) and pull (row, pulldown, chinup); in Workout 3 it will be a kettlebell swing, glute bridge, or stepup. (Don't worry if you don't know what all those exercises are. You will soon enough.)

The next group includes your complementary exercises. The structure is the same: a lower-body exercise (usually a lunge or carry), a push, and a pull. The upper-body exercises will, as advertised, complement the ones you do in the first group. So if your primary push is a shoulder press, you'll do a pushup or chest-press variation as your complementary exercise. Same with the pull: If your primary exercise is a chinup or lat pulldown, you'll complement that with a row.

In Workout 3, you'll do a pair of accessory exercises—one each for your triceps and biceps—as your push and pull.

The biggest difference between primary and complementary/accessory exercises is how you do them. You do the primary exercises with the goal of generating increasing levels of mechanical tension. You're training for strength, not demonstrating it. If the final set calls for 5 reps, you want to finish it with the sense that you could have done one more, knowing you'll come back next week and do it again, this time with a heavier weight. When you can't increase the weight, you move on to a different set of primary exercises and repeat the process.

You do the complementary and accessory exercises with the goal of inducing a deeper level of muscular exhaustion. You're going for metabolic stress and muscle damage, both powerful hypertrophy mechanisms. Of course, you still want to get stronger from week to week on your complementary exercises, but now it's okay to push your muscles to what feels like their limit. In fact, it's *necessary*. You want your muscles to shake, and to feel engorged with blood.

Another way to look at it: When you do the primary exercises, you're *training*; when you do the complementary and accessory exercises, you're *working out*. You're going for long-term adaptations in both parts of the workout, but in the final part you want immediate feedback from your body.

Should You Accessorize?

Now, about that "final part": The Phase One and Two workouts, as written, usually take me about 45 to 50 minutes. (The Phase Three workouts are more like an hour.) Usually, I'm pretty wiped by the end. The last thing I want to do is more exercises. You, on the other hand, may feel like you're just getting your second wind. If that's the case, you probably want to know what else you can do.

My answer is simple and unoriginal: Follow your bliss. If you want to add some exercises for small muscle groups (biceps, triceps, calves, lower epiglottis), go ahead. If you want to add some intervals, or stretches, or anything else, feel free. Just follow these rules.

1. The 80/20 rule. At least 80 percent of your training—that is, 80 percent of your time *and effort*—must be devoted to the actual workout. No more than 20 percent of time or effort can go to accessory exercises or training modalities.

2. The "nothing hurts" rule. This applies to the primary and complementary exercises as well. There's probably more risk with those, since you're using heavier weights and doing more complex lifts. But sometimes we take our most foolish risks with the exercises that seem simplest. (See "Safety First!" on page 160 for more.)

3. The balance rule. Never do an extra push exercise without also doing a pull. (It's okay to do a pull without a push, however; I've never heard of imbalances or complications arising from extra pulls.) And never train your biceps without equal work for your triceps. You don't necessarily have to achieve balance each day. Just aim for it within a week's workouts.

4. The multitasking rule. It's not really a rule so much as a decent idea: Try to do more than one thing with each exercise. For example, if you do an arm exercise with one arm at a time, or in a kneeling or half-kneeling position, you add a core-stability challenge. Working one limb at a time also doubles the volume of the exercise, which can add a conditioning challenge if you're working at a fast pace.

All That Other Stuff You Like to Do

The question I hear most often from readers is some variation on "How do I incorporate . . . ?" or "On the days in between workouts, can I . . . . ? " I wish I had a simple answer. In a vacuum, everything is good and more is often better, especially when the goal is fat loss. But in the context of your own body and your own program, who knows?

Take running, for example. Great form of exercise. Great sport. Great, that is, for runners. Anecdotally, I think all of us know novice runners who tried it for weight loss and ended up gaining a few pounds, either because of an injury that left them unable to exercise at all, or because their appetite overcompensated for the sudden challenge to their energy reserves.

As an adjunct to the Lean Muscle Plan, running should work as well as any other supplemental exercise, as long as you have experience and know your body can handle it. The impact on your joints can interfere with your recovery from strength training, even if it doesn't lead to injury.

That's the key to any exercise you do in conjunction with an aggressive lifting program: It helps only if it allows full recovery from one workout to the next. How do you judge recovery?

▶ You get stronger from week to week.

▶ You develop better form on key exercises like squats and dead-lifts, due to improved mobility in your ankles and hips and bet-ter stability in your core and shoulders.

▶ You don't experience lingering soreness in your muscles or joints; increasing joint soreness over time means you're doing more harm than good. This also applies to any accessory exer-cises you tack on at the end of the workouts.

▶ You look forward to your workouts and have plenty of energy for them; you sometimes have to hold yourself back to keep from pushing too hard.

SAFETY FIRST!

INJURIES ARE A TAX ON PEOPLE WHO DON'T PAY ATTENTION

My younger daughter, when she was 9, suffered a broken leg when the golf cart she was driving rolled over and fell on top of her. I assume you're now thinking one or more of these thoughts.

1. "A 9-year-old was driving a *golf cart*? Are you the worst parent *on earth*?"
2. "Damn! Lucky it was just a leg and not something worse!"
3. "Seriously, are you the worst f***ing parent *on earth*?"

The parental negligence, I agree, was staggering. It's mitigated only by the facts that (a) the golf cart wasn't ours; (b) the people who owned it had no idea their older children had talked our youngest into driving it; and (c) the adults were all out of sight when our daughter took the wheel.

Now suppose you were working in the emergency room when we came in with our daughter. How would you classify this injury? Since it involved a golf cart, would you record it as golf-related? The answer is kind of relevant. When we talk about weight-room safety, we typically use data from emergency-room visits. And with those, it's hard to separate injuries that occurred while lifting from those that merely involved lifting equipment.

In one review of this data, 38 percent of visits linked to strength training happened to teenagers. Hands and feet were the most frequent injury sites. Since weight-room injuries are an overwhelmingly male phenomenon, and since testosterone-addled teenage boys aren't known for their caution, who knows if the knuckleheads who crushed their pinkies or dropped weights on their metatarsals were actually training? They might've been playing Frisbee golf with 10-pound plates.

SPECIAL TOPIC

For adult lifters, the most common injury site is the torso. The older you are, the more likely it is that any lifting-related emergency-room visit will be for a joint injury or muscle tear. That's some serious pain, with potentially long-term consequences, and brings up perhaps the most fundamental safety tip of all.

Treat every weight as if it's heavy.

Bad things happen when you let your guard down. You don't want to be the guy who goes through life complaining of a bad back because of one moment in the gym when he lost focus.

Even the accidents caused by someone else—the idiot who drops a weight on your foot, for example—are sometimes avoided when you exercise some caution. This is one reason why I'm down on iPods in the gym. They don't just tune out distractions—they also tune out things you should actually notice, like potential dangers.

When you treat every weight as if it's heavy, no matter who's lifting it, you virtually eliminate one category of injuries: the ones you get from not paying attention.

Oh, and please don't let your children drive golf carts. There's only one way it could end well, and many ways it couldn't.

CHAPTER 10:

THE WARMUP

THIS IS THE PART OF THE PROGRAM that's most conducive to individual tinkering. The longer you lift, and the better you understand your own body, the better your warmup should work. I rarely do the exact same warmup routine twice in one week. Instead, I mix things up based on which muscles and joints feel tighter than normal. And of course, "normal" is a moving target, thanks to my on-again, off-again battles with knee and hip problems.

You may want to add a few minutes of general warmup before starting these exercises. A general warmup is most useful if you work out in the morning, especially in the colder times of year. It doesn't have to be anything fancy. A few minutes on a treadmill or exercise bike, some jumping jacks, or a little shadow boxing should do the trick. You may also want to add some foam-rolling exercises or stretches.

If I may go below the belt for a moment: Your warmup is to your workout as foreplay is to lovemaking. It's not wrong if it works.

The goal of the following exercises is to mobilize your hip and shoulder joints and activate key muscles surrounding those joints. That should take about 10 minutes—less if you're already familiar and comfortable with them, more if they're new to you. Again, whatever you do is only wrong if:

▶ It doesn't properly prepare your body for the rest of the workout

▶ It wears you out before you start lifting

You know you've hit the sweet spot if you break a light sweat, and you can't wait to move some iron.

1. THREE-POINT SHOULDER ROTATION

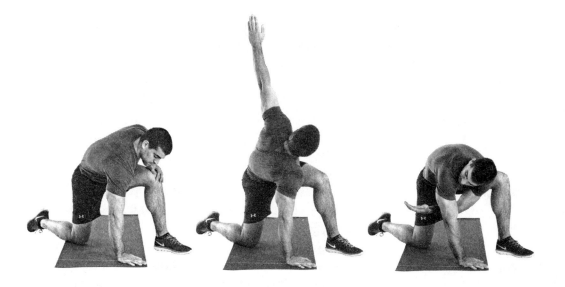

We start with the shoulders—or, more accurately, the thoracic spine. The better your thoracic mobility, the easier it should be to safely stabilize your lumbar spine.

Assume the position: Start in the half-kneeling position, with your right knee down and left foot forward. (If you aren't on a padded or carpeted floor, you'll want to put a towel or pad beneath your knee.) Both knees are bent about 90 degrees. Bend forward from the hips so your torso is parallel to the floor, and place your right hand on the floor directly beneath your right shoulder and in line with your left foot.

Move:

1. Rotate your upper torso as you reach up and back with your left hand. Follow your hand with your eyes. Both arms are now perpendicular to the floor.

2. Reverse the movement, pulling your left arm down. Reach behind your right arm and past your torso. That's 1 rep.

Do 8 reps, then switch sides and repeat.

2. ROCKING HIP FLEXOR MOBILIZATION

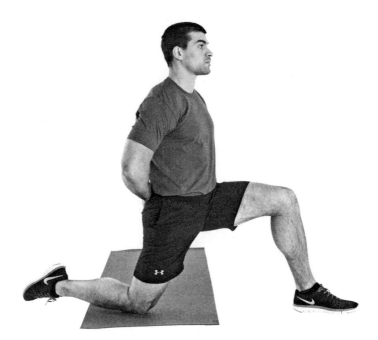

Now we start the multistage process of making sure your hip muscles are activated and ready to work through their ideal range of motion. We'll start with the hip flexors, the strips of muscle on the front of your pelvis, which get short and weak from hours of sitting every day. You'll simultaneously engage your glute muscles.

Assume the position: Start again in the half-kneeling position—right knee and left foot on the floor. This time, keep your torso upright, with your hands behind your back.

Move:

1. Squeeze your right glute muscle, and shift your hips forward.

2. Feel the stretch down the right side of your pelvis and the top of your right thigh.

3. Relax and return to the starting position.

Do 6 reps, then switch sides and repeat.

SPIDERMAN WITH REACH

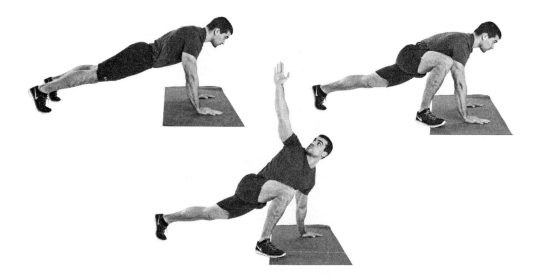

This exercise, which I use almost every workout, combines a good hip flexor stretch with shoulder rotation, and throws in a mild core-stability challenge. You can do it after the two previous exercises, or as an alternative to them to save time.

Assume the position: Get into pushup position, with your hands on the floor directly below your shoulders, your toes about hip-width apart, and your body in a straight line from your neck through your ankles.

Move:

1. Without lifting your torso, lift your right foot up next to your right hand.

2. Drop your hips *slightly* and feel a stretch in the hip flexors on your right.

3. Reach up and back with your right hand as you rotate your shoulders to the right. Follow your hand with your eyes.

4. Return to the pushup position.

5. Repeat to the other side.

Do 5 or 6 reps to each side.

3. GLUTE BRIDGE

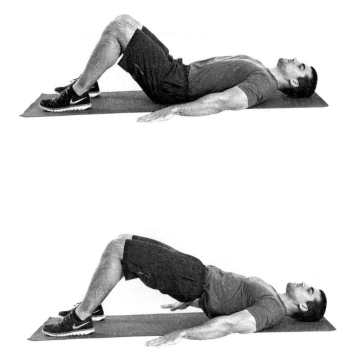

This is the simplest activation exercise for your gluteus maximus, the biggest, strongest muscle in your body.

Assume the position: Lie faceup on the floor, with your knees bent, feet on the floor, and arms out to your sides.

Move:

1. Push down through your heels to lift your hips off the floor until your body forms a straight line from shoulders to knees.

2. Hold for 2 seconds, feeling the contraction primarily in your glutes and secondarily in your hamstrings; you shouldn't feel any discomfort in your lower back.

3. Lower your hips toward the floor, stopping just before they touch, and repeat.

Do 10 to 15 reps.

ADVANCED OPTION:

COOK HIP LIFT

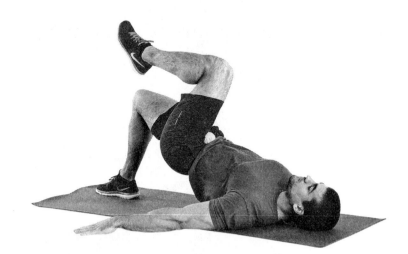

You'll need a tennis ball to do this challenging single-leg variation on the glute bridge, which is named for physical therapist Gray Cook. By activating your hip flexors to hold the tennis ball in place against your lower abdomen, you take your lower-back muscles out of the movement. This ensures that your glutes and hamstrings do all the work.

Assume the position: Set up as you did for the glute bridge, but place a tennis ball on the left side of your lower abs, just below your bottom rib. Lift your left knee toward your chest, squeezing the ball between your upper thigh and abdomen.

Move:

1. Push down through your right heel and lift your hips, as described above, while holding the ball in place with your left leg.

2. Lower your hips and repeat.

Do 5 to 10 reps on each side. The first few are the hardest; it may take you a couple workouts to even work up to 5 reps per side.

MORE STRENUOUS ALTERNATIVE:

SWISS BALL HIP LIFT WITH LEG CURL

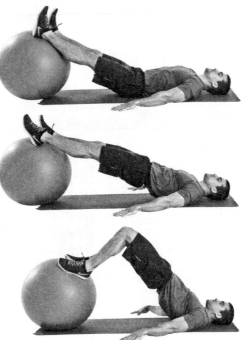

This one works the glutes, hamstrings, and calves. You can use it as a complementary exercise in the strength program if you like it and find it challenging in the range of 10 to 15 reps.

Assume the position: Grab a Swiss ball and lie on your back on the floor, with your heels on the ball and arms out to your sides for balance.

Move:

1. Lift your hips so your body is straight from shoulders to ankles.

2. Bend your knees to pull the ball toward you, lifting your body until your knees are bent 90 degrees, your feet are flat on the ball, and your body forms a line from your shoulders to your knees.

3. Hold that position for 1 or 2 seconds, feeling the contraction.

4. Roll the ball back as you straighten your legs and lower your body, stopping just before your hips touch the floor.

Do 8 to 10 reps.

4. BAND-RESISTED CLAM

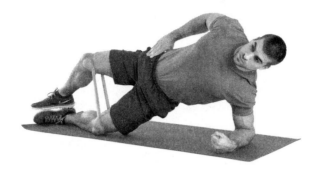

This exercise develops hip abduction strength, which is something the average guy would never think is important enough to train. I didn't think it was important either, until I learned that knee pain often originates in the hips. Strengthening those muscles should contribute to improved strength and power in the gym and more speed outside of it.

You'll need an elastic band that's pliable enough to let you spread your knees wide apart, but firm enough so it's challenging to hold that position. I highly recommend purchasing your own from Perform Better (performbetter.com). They're 9 inches long and 2 inches wide, and cost just a couple bucks each.

Assume the position: Take the band and put it around your thighs, just above your knees. Lie on your side on the floor, with your knees bent about 90 degrees and your hips bent about 45 degrees. (Your thighs and torso will form a 135-degree angle.) Set your forearm on the floor to support your upper body.

Move:

1. Spread your knees as far apart as you can, keeping your bottom leg on the floor and the sides of your feet touching each other.

2. Hold that position 30 to 60 seconds, then switch sides and repeat.

Start with a band that allows you to hold for 30 seconds per side. When you can hold for 60 seconds per side with that band, move up to a more challenging band.

5. BODY-WEIGHT SQUAT

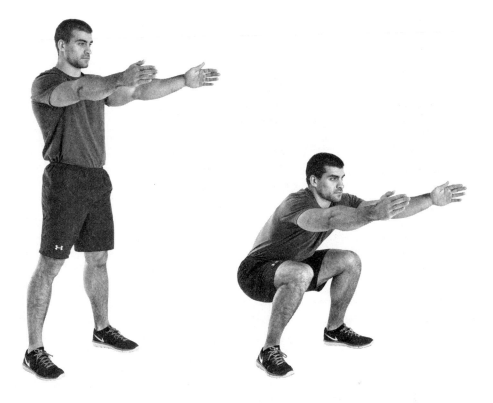

Now that your glutes have been activated, and mildly tested by the band-resisted clam, you're ready to squat with the full range of motion and perfect form.

Assume the position: Stand with your feet shoulder-width apart, toes pointed forward, and arms straight out in front of you.

Move:

1. Push your hips straight back, as if you were aiming them toward a chair.

2. Descend until your upper thighs are parallel to the floor.

3. Return to the starting position, with your knees and hips following the exact same path they used on the way down.

Do 10 to 15 reps.

6. TRIPLE LUNGE

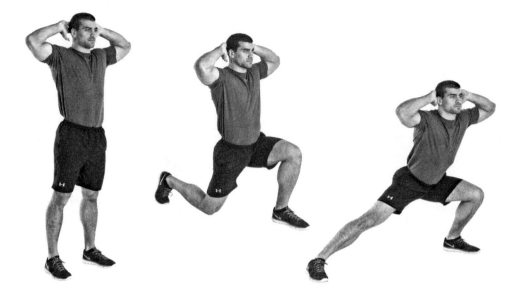

Assume the position: Stand with your feet hip-width apart and your hands behind your head in the prisoner grip.

Move:

1. Step forward with your left leg, lowering your body until both knees are bent about 90 degrees. Keep your torso upright. Step back to the starting position.

2. Take a long step to your left, descending into a deep side lunge, with your left knee bent and your chest over your left thigh. Your right leg should be straight, with both feet flat on the floor and parallel to each other.

3. Push back to the starting position.

4. Step back with your left leg, descending until your left knee nearly touches the floor. As with the forward lunge, keep your body upright. Step back to the starting position.

5. Repeat the lunge sequence—forward, side, back—with your right leg.

Do 2 or 3 triple lunges with each leg. You don't want to exhaust your muscles, just prepare them to be exhausted.

7. SINGLE-LEG ROMANIAN DEADLIFT

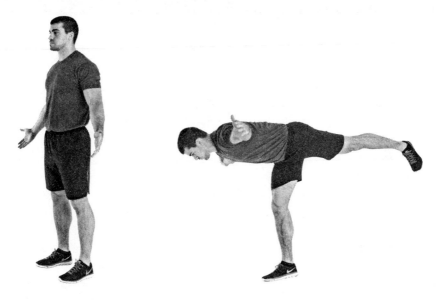

You'll see the single-leg RDL done with dumbbells or a barbell. But I've always liked it better as a warmup. It tests your balance, opens up your chest, and streches the hamstrings of the working leg, followed by a contraction of your glutes to return to the starting position.

Assume the position: Stand with your feet hip-width apart, arms at your sides, palms facing forward, thumbs out.

Move:

1. Slide your left leg back as you bend forward at the hips and raise your arms straight out to the sides. Your leg and torso should move as a unit, keeping the same alignment until both are parallel to the floor and perpendicular to your right leg.

2. Feel the stretch through your right hamstring, and squeeze the muscles in your upper back to open up your chest and shoulders.

3. Fire your right glute muscles to return to the starting position.

4. As your left toes touch the floor, sweep your leg back to begin the next repetition.

Do 5 to 8 reps with each leg. Practice the move without exhausting the muscles.

CHAPTER 11

CORE TRAINING

AT THE END OF CHAPTER 4, I explained why I don't like the saying "Abs are made in the kitchen," one of the fitness world's most popular clichés. I had abs as a teenager, decades before I had a clue about healthy nutrition. I would have preferred biceps and deltoids, but abs were my reward for all the enthusiastic training I did in my youth, including hundreds and hundreds of situps.

I don't do situps on a regular basis anymore, based on the persuasive research of Stuart McGill, PhD, a professor of spine biomechanics at the University of Waterloo in Ontario. He believes the repeated stress to your lower back is an injurious mechanism. As he wrote in *Low Back Disorders,* his first book: "Those who are training for health never need to perform a situp; those training for performance may get better results by judiciously incorporating them into their routine."

He's not saying everyone who does situps will get injured, and it doesn't mean you should never do this exercise, ever. It just means the risk of doing them frequently and chronically is unacceptable for most of us.

Risk, of course, is relative. The longer you train, the stronger you get; and the more adaptations your body makes, the harder it's going to be to get even stronger, and to make more advanced adaptations. That may be the best reason to take core training seriously: It enhances your ability to do everything else more aggressively, with fewer injuries.

With that out of the way, let's . . .

I'm sorry, what's that? You want to know the best exercises to get ripped abs? Okay, you're right. We should talk about that before we get into the core-training program.

Ab-Ripping 101

Fitness pros see questions like this pretty much every day. If you think it's a reasonable question to ask, I guarantee you won't like the answer. Which is: When someone tells you he has a unique exercise, diet, or combined program to produce a specific visual or aesthetic outcome, that person *is lying out his ass.*

The shape of your muscles is out of your control; no workout can give you a six-pack (not to mention an eight-pack) unless that's in your genetic blueprint. Where your body deposits fat is also out of your control, which means there's no way to target specific areas for rapid or selective fat loss. The subcutaneous fat around your midsection might come off fast or slow. It might come off right away, before you lose fat in other areas. Or it might not come off until you've lost fat everywhere else, leaving you so emaciated you make Sid Vicious look healthy and well-nourished.

None of this means you're defenseless against your genetics. I like this quote from my friend Nick Tumminello: "You can't spot-reduce, but you can spot-*enhance.*" Wider shoulders make your waist seem smaller. Adding muscle to your glutes and thighs makes you appear more athletic and powerful. And, yes, adding some size to your mid-body muscles, all else being equal, should help you look leaner, stronger, and more powerfully athletic.

But I don't want to imply that's an automatic benefit of the following core-training exercises. I see it as more of a side effect, a part of the process that leads you to a better physique than you have now. To quote Nick one more time: "Core exercises don't have direct carryover to performance. They strengthen links in the chain, allowing the chain to produce more force." More force production means more muscle development; more muscle development means more productive workouts and a slightly faster metabolism, both of which help you get leaner than you are now.

Put another way, when your body can *do* more, you can *be* more.

How the Program Works

The core exercises are divided into three categories, which I explained in Chapter 3.

Stability

These are static exercises in which you hold a challenging position for a designated amount of time. You'll do these in your first workout each week, which will typically be the one most focused on developing maximum strength.

Dynamic Stability

In these exercises you'll hold a stable position while moving your arms or legs. You'll do them in your second workout of the week, which will typically be the most hypertrophy-focused workout.

Strength and Hypertrophy

These are the most strenuous core exercises, which is why you'll do them in the third and final workout each week. In that workout you'll typically use lighter weights for your strength exercises, and either move faster or do more total work.

You'll find three progressive phases of exercises in the three categories of this program. In each category you want to start with the basic exercises, and move up when you master them—you hit the maximum time for stability exercises, max reps for dynamic stability, or a performance limit on the strength and hypertrophy exercises. You might max out on all the basic exercises your first couple of weeks on the Lean Muscle Plan, and that's fine. Just make sure you pass each test before moving on to the next challenge.

STABILITY EXERCISES

PHASE ONE

PLANK

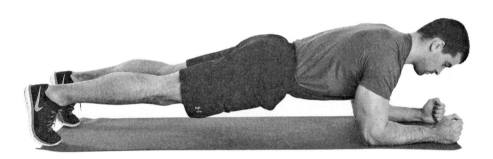

I present to you the most boring exercise in human history. It's the fitness equivalent of a box spring—the least interesting part of your bed, but the one that ensures a good night's sleep. (Unless you have a memory-foam mattress or a European-style platform bed, in which case you don't need a box spring, and the comparison doesn't work.) The basic plank is an *anti-extension* exercise. It trains your core muscles to keep your lower back and pelvis locked in the neutral position, which means your lumbar spine retains its natural arch. Your core muscles need to work together to prevent your back from extending into a deeper arch, which is potentially injurious. The plank develops endurance in those muscles, setting you up for success in pretty much everything you do in the weight room.

Assume the position: Get down on the floor in a modified pushup position, with your weight resting on your forearms and toes, and your body in a straight line from neck to ankles. You probably want to put a pad beneath your forearms if you aren't on a padded or carpeted floor. Don't deliberately flex or brace anything. Just hold your body in that alignment.

Hold for up to 60 seconds per set. When you can maintain the plank for two 1-minute sets, move on to more challenging versions.

SIDE PLANK

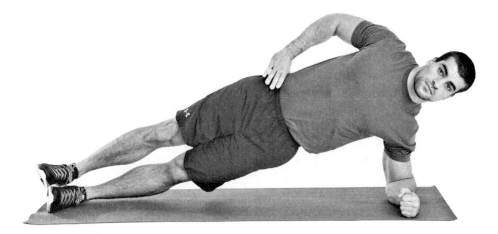

This is a not-boring exercise, mostly because it's more challenging than you think it will be, especially if you haven't done it in a while. It'll expose weaknesses and imbalances you didn't know you had.

Assume the position: Get on the floor with your weight resting on your left forearm and the outside edge of your left foot. (Make sure you set your forearm on a pad.) Stack your right foot on top of your left, and lift your body so it forms a straight line from your nose through the midline of your body. Rest your right hand on your right hip.

Hold for up to 30 seconds, then switch sides and repeat.

You can easily tweak these exercises to make them a bit harder.

Elevate your feet, *using a box or step. This works for either exercise.*

Reduce the base of support. *Lift one arm or leg off the floor for the plank. You can hold for 30 seconds with each limb elevated. For the side plank, a super-challenging variation is to lift your bottom leg off the floor, then bend your knee and tuck your foot against the underside of your top leg, as shown below. This means your weight is supported by your forearm and the inside edge of your top foot.*

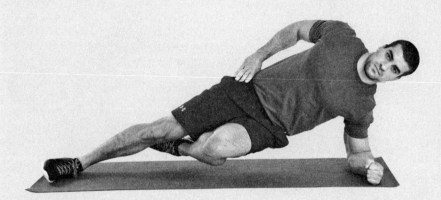

Add an element of instability. *Do the plank with your forearms on a Swiss ball, or with your feet in a pair of suspension straps. (The TRX and Jungle Gym are the best-known brands.) You can also elevate your feet in a suspension system for the side plank—fair warning, this is a real ass-kicker.*

LONG-LEVER PLANK

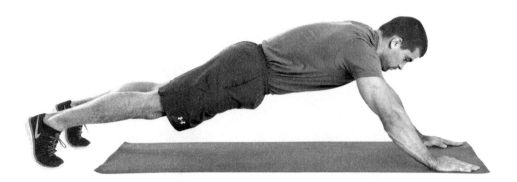

The basic plank offers a modest challenge to the muscles of your abdomen and lower back. This extended remix challenges everything from your shoulders to your ankles.

Assume the position: Get into pushup position, with your hands directly below your shoulders and weight resting on your hands and toes. Set your body in a straight line from neck to ankles. Now walk your hands forward 6 to 12 inches, or even a bit farther if you can keep your lower back and pelvis in the neutral position.

Hold the extended position for 30 seconds, then walk your hands back to the pushup position. Relax, catch your breath, and repeat.

You can tweak the long-lever plank the same ways you tweaked the basic version.

Place your feet on a Swiss ball.

Put your feet in a suspension system.

Place your hands on unstable objects, *like a pair of medicine balls or the handles of a suspension system.*

Add chest taps (shown). *Hold the basic position for 5 seconds, then slowly lift your left hand and tap your right shoulder. Return to the starting position, then repeat with your right hand.*

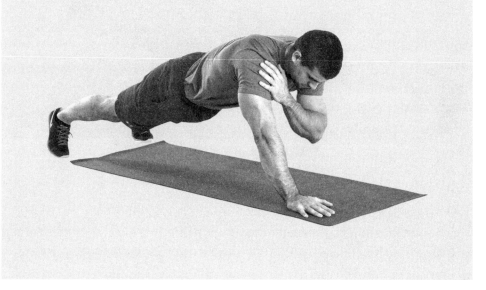

CONTRALATERAL CORE LIFT

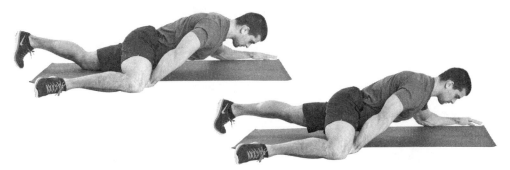

I learned this exercise from my friend Chad Waterbury. It's adapted from an exercise system called dynamic neuromuscular stabilization (DNS), which aims for coordinated control of almost all your body's muscles. This particular exercise develops the link between your shoulder and opposite-side hip, with your core acting as the conduit for that force transfer.

Assume the position: The setup is a bit more complicated.

1. Lie facedown with your left leg straight and right leg bent at the hip and knee so your right thigh is perpendicular to your torso.

2. Your left arm is on the floor, with the upper arm perpendicular to your torso, elbow bent, and hand even with your left ear.

3. Grab the inside of your right thigh with your right hand.

4. Lift your head an inch or two off the floor, and tuck your chin.

5. Now comes the actual exercise: Push yourself up off the floor, with your weight supported by your right knee and left elbow. Your left knee is still on the floor, but it's not supporting much of your weight.

Hold for 5 seconds, forcing at least one breath in and out (which won't be easy). Switch sides and repeat. Do 3 or 4 reps on each side. Work up to 30-second holds, forcing a breath in and out every few seconds.

NEED A BIGGER CHALLENGE?

Make it even tougher by lifting your left knee off the floor (bottom photo), further reducing your base of support.

PHASE ONE

DEAD BUG 1

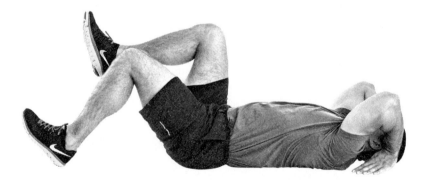

The dead bug is another anti-extension exercise, but one that targets different muscles. Whereas the plank offers a mild challenge to the abdominal and lower-back muscles, the more advanced versions of the dead bug offer a *serious* challenge to the rectus abdominis (the six-pack muscle), obliques, and hip flexors.

I've seen so many versions of the dead bug, and so many different variations on the exercise name (dying bug, resurrected dead bug), that it's hard to choose which one to start with, or which progressions to include. I ended up with three. Everyone should start with dead bug 1. If the first set is easy, do the next set with dead bug 2. That one shouldn't be easy. Not for anyone. Not if you're doing it as described, with a deliberate pace and full range of motion. If you hit the maximum reps, feel good about yourself for a week. Then come back next week and try dead bug 3, which, as you'll see, is as challenging as you want to make it.

Assume the position: Lie on your back, perpendicular to a wall, with your hands touching the wall behind your head. (No wall? You can place your hands on the floor, as shown here.) Start with your legs up in the air and knees bent. Push your lower back into the floor, and then press your hands into the wall behind you. You should feel your abs and lats engaged to hold you in this position.

Work:

1. Lower your left heel to the floor, keeping your knee bent. Raise it back to the starting position.

2. Same thing with your right leg: Lower, touch your heel to the floor, raise it. Do the entire movement at a steady, controlled speed. You should feel your core muscles working continuously.

Do 2 sets of 10 to 12 reps with each leg.

DEAD BUG 2

From the same starting position, straighten your right leg as you lower it, and touch the back of your leg to the floor. Return to the starting position, and repeat with your left leg. Again, use a steady, controlled speed, and keep your lower back pressed to the floor.

Do 2 sets of 10 to 12 reps with each leg.

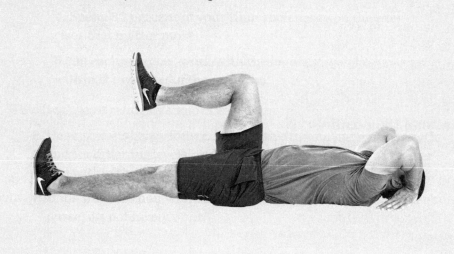

DEAD BUG 3

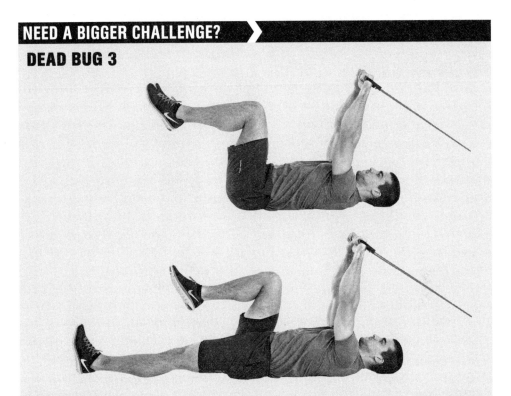

Even though it's impossible to judge how intensely your muscles are working, my abdominals feel like they're 100 percent engaged when I do this variation I learned from strength coach Mike Robertson.

1. Take a band and loop it around something solid, like the base of a squat rack.

2. Grab the ends of the band and position yourself on the floor with your arms straight up over your chest. There should be enough tension in the band so you feel your core muscles working hard just to hold this position.

3. Raise your legs, with your knees bent, and push your lower back into the floor.

4. Now comes the hard part: Extend your right leg and touch the back of it to the floor. Return to the starting position and repeat with your left. Stop the set if you feel your lower back start to rise off the floor.

Do 2 sets of 8 to 10 reps with each leg.

PALLOF PRESS

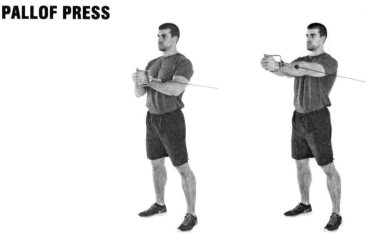

You need to be able to rotate your torso; virtually every sport we play involves some kind of twist. But the rotation has to occur at your shoulders and hips. The big, thick vertebrae of your lower back have a very short range of motion, just a degree or two in each direction. That's where *anti-rotation exercises* like the Pallof press—invented by physical therapist John Pallof—come into play.

Assume the position: Attach a D-shaped handle to a cable pulley and set it to chest height. (You can also use a band.) Grab the handle with both hands and step out until you have tension in the cable. Stand sideways to the machine in an athletic position—feet shoulder-width apart, toes pointed forward, knees bent slightly, chest up, shoulders down, core tight, eyes focused straight ahead—holding the handle against your chest.

Work:

1. Push the handle straight out from your chest until your arms are straight.

2. Hold that position for a count of 2. You should feel the torso and hip muscles on the side farthest from the machine working to keep you upright.

3. Pull the handle back to your chest, and repeat.

4. Do all your reps, then turn around and repeat facing the opposite direction.

Do 2 sets of 8 to 10 reps to each side.

Static hold: *Instead of pushing the handle out and back, hold it in front of your chest with your arms straight.*

Hold for up to 30 seconds; do 2 sets per side.

Pallof 2.0: *This and the next one come from Nick Tumminello. It starts off like the static hold, with the handle straight out in front of your chest. Now, keeping your arms straight, move your hands from side to side along a very short path—about 12 to 18 inches, stopping at the outer edges of your chest. Keep your hips facing forward, with all the rotation coming from your shoulders.*

Do 2 sets of 15 to 20 reps per side.

Lateral Pallof press: *Start in the half-kneeling position, as shown below, with the knee farthest from the machine on the floor and your torso upright. With the handle against your chest, push it up over your head. The challenge here is to prevent your torso from bending laterally toward the machine. Hold at the top for 2 seconds.*

Do 2 sets of 4 to 6 reps per side.

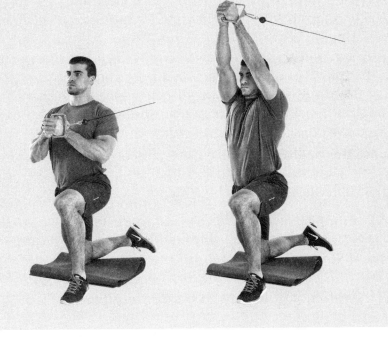

SWISS BALL ROLLOUT

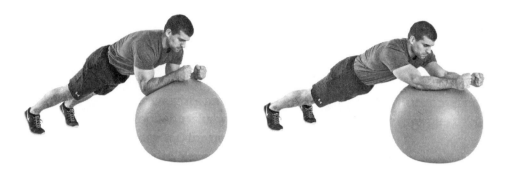

This is the ultimate anti-extension exercise. In one recent study comparing 10 different core exercises, the rollout crushed the others for activation of the upper part of the rectus abdominis, the six-pack muscle. It also gave a significant challenge to the lower rectus and obliques. It could very well be the single most effective core exercise in the Lean Muscle Plan, in terms of building muscle and burning calories. Consequently, it was rated among the toughest exercises to perform in that study.

If you try the exercise and realize you aren't ready for it, there's no reason to feel bad about yourself. It's not a sign of low testosterone or poor character. It just means your core muscles don't yet have the strength and coordination to stabilize your spine in an advanced exercise. The worst thing you can do is labor through it with poor form.

Assume the position: Get into plank position with your forearms on a Swiss ball and your toes on the floor. The farther apart you set your feet, the easier the exercise should be.

Work:

1. Roll the ball forward by straightening your arms and pushing the ball forward while keeping your lower back and pelvis locked in the neutral position.

2. Pull the ball back to the starting position, and repeat.

Do 2 sets of 6 to 8 reps.

AB-WHEEL ROLLOUT

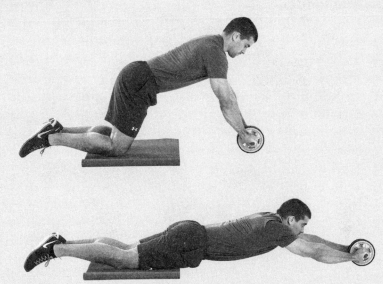

The range of motion on the Swiss ball rollout is short, while the execution is complicated because the ball can roll in any direction. You invest some energy in preventing lateral movement. The ab-wheel rollout solves both problems, assuming you have access to one. (You can pick one up online or in a sporting goods store for $10 to $15.)

Assume the position: Unless you're a gymnast, you'll do this exercise from your knees. Kneel on a pad with your torso bent forward at the hips. Hold the wheel's handles with your arms straight and perpendicular to the floor.

Work:

1. Roll forward as far as you can while keeping a neutral spine.

2. Pull the wheel back to the starting position, again finishing with a neutral spine; you don't need to flex your torso forward; multiple studies have shown tremendous ab-muscle activation with the form I just described.

Do 2 sets of 6 to 8 reps.

SWISS BALL JACKKNIFE

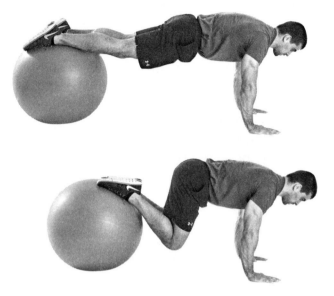

The second Phase Three core exercise will directly challenge your hip flexors, while forcing the rest of your core muscles to work moderately hard to keep your back in the neutral position.

Assume the position: Get into the pushup position with your shins on top of the ball and your hands on the floor, directly beneath your shoulders. Set your body in a (nearly) straight line from neck to ankles.

Work:

1. Pull your knees toward your chest while keeping your back in the original position.

2. Push back to the starting position and repeat.

Do 2 sets of 6 to 10 reps.

NEED A BIGGER CHALLENGE? ▶

I doubt many of you need a tougher exercise than this one. But if you want to make it more challenging, you can do a pushup after you straighten your legs at the end of each jackknife.

STRENGTH AND HYPERTROPHY EXERCISES

PHASE ONE

MCGILL CURLUP

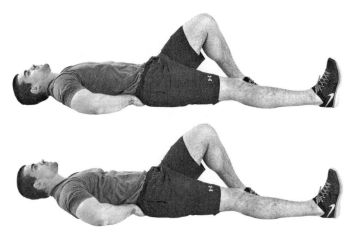

This is Stuart McGill's alternative to situps and crunches. Your back stays in the neutral position, but you still give the rectus abdominis serious work.

Assume the position: Lie on your back on the floor with your right leg straight and left knee bent, with your left foot flat on the floor next to your right knee. Place both hands on the floor palms-down beneath your lower back. Rest your forearms on the floor.

Work:

1. Raise your head and shoulders a couple inches off the floor while keeping your elbows down.

2. Feel the squeeze in your rectus abdominis as you hold for a second or two.

3. Lower your head and shoulders to the floor, and repeat.

Do 2 sets of 6 to 10 reps—1 set with the left knee elevated, the other with the right knee up.

NEED A BIGGER CHALLENGE? ⟩

The curlup, as I noted, isn't a traditional crunch. It's like the difference between a human and a chimpanzee. We share 98 percent of our DNA, but the 2 percent that's different is what moved us to the top of the food chain. You advance not by extending the range of motion or adding external resistance, but by adding internal resistance. You pre-brace your abs—that is, you tighten your muscles, as if flexing in the mirror for a selfie—and then you curl up against that solid wall of resistance. If it's not hard to do (really, really hard), work on your pre-bracing. Once you get it right, you'll know it. A 2-inch range of motion will feel like the toughest core exercise you've ever attempted.

There's actually a way to make it even more challenging: In the top position, force two or three breaths in and out.

HALF TURKISH GETUP

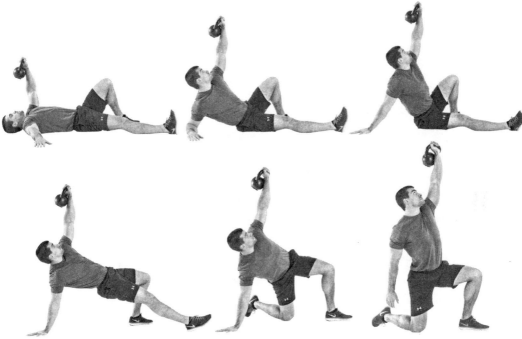

The Turkish getup is a complex movement in which you start flat on your back, holding a weight with one arm over your chest, and rise to a standing position with the weight overhead. I'm not sure where it comes from. One origin story says it was first used by Turkish wrestlers; another says it was a circus-strongman trick that has nothing to do with either Turks or wrestlers. What I question isn't the origin so much as the second half of the exercise, the part where you stand up. It's certainly hard to do, and there's nothing wrong with that. But a few years back, during one of my bouts with knee pain, I realized I could get what I wanted out of the exercise by doing the first half and skipping the part that aggravated my knees. Since then I've seen trainers recommend the half getup for core strength.

Assume the position:

1. Lie on your back on the floor, with a dumbbell or kettlebell next to your left shoulder.

(continued)

2. Grab the weight with both hands and lift it to your chest.

3. Let go with your right hand and raise it straight over your chest with your left arm.

4. Set your left foot on the floor with your left knee bent. Keep your right leg straight; it'll stay flat on the floor throughout the movement.

5. Set your right arm on the floor at roughly a 45-degree angle to your torso.

6. Focus your eyes on the weight; they'll stay on the weight throughout the movement—both up and down.

Work:

1. Push down hard with your left heel and raise your torso off the floor.

2. As you lift your torso, bend your right arm and slide it behind you so your right forearm and elbow now support your upper body.

3. Straighten your right arm and push the weight in your left hand toward the ceiling.

4. Raise your hips off the floor so your body forms a straight line (more or less) from your shoulders to your right ankle.

5. Bend your right leg and slide it back so your right knee rests on the floor and helps support your weight.

6. Lift your right hand off the floor and straighten your torso so your body is in a half-kneeling position.

7. In the full getup, you'd rise to a standing position. And you can do that if you want. But if you have balky knees (like me), or think the exercise is complicated enough as it is (also like me), reverse the sequence and lower your body to the floor.

8. Do all your reps, then switch sides and repeat.

Do 2 or 3 sets of 3 to 5 reps on each side.

PARTIAL DRAGON FLAG

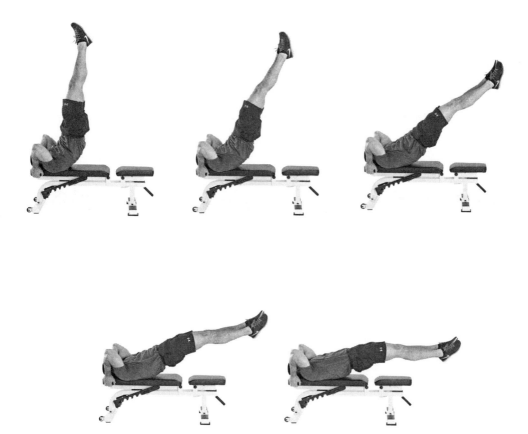

If you can do the full dragon flag, you're awesome, and I should probably be taking advice from you. As far as I know, it was first used by Bruce Lee, and then popularized by the training sequence in *Rocky IV*. But it doesn't matter, because no matter how cool it is (and like all the proto-CrossFit training in *Rocky IV*, it's *very* cool), approximately 0.000001 percent of all adults who can do at least 1 set of crunches will ever be able to do a dragon flag, as shown here. Thus, the adjective: Just doing a partial dragon flag will hit your abs in such a unique and intense way that you'll wonder why you ever thought the crunch was worth a minute of your time.

Assume the position:

Lie on your back on a bench (or any flat surface, as long as you have something sturdy to hold behind you). Grasp the sides of the bench next to your ears. Kick your legs straight up, and lift your torso so all your weight rests on your shoulders (not your neck!). Tighten everything up.

Work:

1. Keeping your hips straight, lower your torso as slowly as you can and as much as you can. Stop when your core asks, in its own special language, "WTF are you trying to do to me?"

2. Drop your hips to the bench, then kick your legs back up and start the next rep.

NEED TO DIAL IT BACK?

1. You can bend your knees to make it a bit easier, but never bend your hips.

2. You probably want to do this without shoes, especially the first few times.

CHAPTER 12:

THE TRAINING PROGRAM

HE LEAN MUSCLE PLAN has three phases. Each phase includes three workouts. To keep it simple, I've labeled them Workout 1, Workout 2, and Workout 3. You want to do each workout once per week, like this.

	MON	TUES	WED	THURS	FRI	SAT	SUN
WEEK 1	Workout 1	Off	Workout 2	Off	Workout 3	Off	Off
WEEK 2	Workout 1	Off	Workout 2	Off	Workout 3	Off	Off
WEEK 3	Workout 1	Off	Workout 2	Off	Workout 3	Off	Off
WEEK 4	Workout 1	Off	Workout 2	Off	Workout 3	Off	Off

Or you can do them Tuesday, Thursday, and Saturday. What matters is that you do the workouts in numerical order, and that you give yourself about 48 hours to recover from each workout. That's when the fun stuff—the tissue remodeling that gives you bigger, stronger muscles—happens.

Most of you should be ready to move from Phase One to Phase Two after 4 weeks. But you don't have to. If you're still improving from week to week—you're using heavier weights, or getting more reps with the same weights—there's no reason to stop. The goal is to avoid Groundhog Day workouts: the exact same exercises, with the exact same weights, with the exact same sets and reps, week after week. When one week's workouts are no better than the previous week's, it's time to change.

Before You Look at the Workouts . . .

Some of you will look at the charts on the following pages (or screens) and know exactly what the program is and how to do it. But most of you won't. When you see "squat" in the first workout, you'll want to ask, "*Which* squat?" It's a complicated question; I answer at length in Chapter 13. Same with "deadlift" and "bench press," among others.

And those are just the primary exercises. When you get to the complementary and accessory exercises, like "lunge" and "cable row," you'll find more ambiguity. At the end of Workout 3, the final two exercises are labeled "biceps curl" and "triceps extension," without specifying which type of curl and extension. You'll find the explanations in Chapter 14.

In each exercise category, I give you what I think is the best choice to start with. You may quickly max out on it, but at least you know you're ready for a more advanced version. The alternative is to jump right into the more technically challenging exercises, which is almost always a bad idea.

Why You Need to Keep a Training Log

I've been using the same system for tracking workouts—printed log pages on a clipboard—for at least a dozen years, maybe longer. Others use spiral notebooks, or higher-tech options like their smartphones. Anything can work. What doesn't work is no log at all. You're doing three different workouts each week, each with at least seven different exercises. Nobody can remember all that without writing it down.

A good training log allows you to track these variables.

Exercise choices. You have a lot of them in the Lean Muscle Plan. Technically, a pushup is a pushup, but when you have dozens of variations, you want to remember which one you did.

Equipment. One exercise can feel completely different, depending on the equipment you use. It could be a barbell, dumbbell(s), kettlebell(s), cable machine, resistance band, suspension system, sandbag, or weight vest. You also have choices within each category. With a cable system, for example, you have straight or angled bars, and single or double handles. The cable machine also gives you a variety of attachment points—high, medium, low, and quite a few in between.

Grip. When using a barbell, a chinup bar, or a straight bar on a cable machine, you can choose wide, medium, or narrow grips, as well as underhand or overhand.

Weight selected. This category is obviously important for tracking progress. You can't trust your memory, especially in the Phase Two and Three workouts, when you're using different weights for almost every set of your primary exercises.

Sometimes you do an exercise with just your body weight. I'll write "BW" in that column on my log; you might have a better code. Just make sure you record it.

Sets and reps. Increasing load isn't the only way to make progress in the weight room. If you go from 8 to 10 reps with the same weight, that's progress. Same if you go from 2 to 3 sets. It's an improvement, and you want to keep an accurate record.

And keep in mind . . . You probably want to record the date of each workout. I also try to track how much time I spend training each day. When a workout that normally takes 50 minutes is finished after 45, I'll check to make sure I didn't forget anything. If it goes past 60 minutes, I know I either maxed something out, requiring more rest between sets, or I spent too much time chatting.

I also use my log to write down which locker I used. I've learned the hard way not to count on my memory for that.

Two Things I No Longer Get Specific About

In some books—including a couple of mine—you'll find directions for the speed of every lift and the amount of time to rest between sets. I got away from that when I realized two things: (1) It was too much to track for many readers; and (2) I rarely paid attention to tempo or rest in my own workouts.

With the heaviest weights, I don't think there's any point in telling you how fast to lift. You lift as fast as you can, and you lower the weights carefully. If anything, stopping to count the seconds might take your mind off your form, which is what matters most for both safety and performance.

Tracking rest is probably most useful to two types of lifters. There's the guy like me, who tends to get impatient between sets. I'll sometimes compromise performance by starting the next set before I'm fully recovered from the last one. Then there's the guy who's easily distracted and takes too much time. That reduces the cumulative fatigue of the training session, which possibly compromises the overall conditioning effect.

So if you need a general guideline, it would go something like this.

On your heaviest sets—6 or fewer reps—rest at least 2 minutes between sets to allow for full recovery. This applies even when you're alternating exercises, which I'll explain in the next section.

▶ On medium-heavy sets—8 to 10 reps—rest about a minute between sets.

▶ When using more than 10 reps, I like to move as quickly as I can from set to set and exercise to exercise. That's the closest I ever get to cardio training.

PHASE ONE

WORKOUT 1

EXERCISE	SETS	REPS
CORE TRAINING: STABILITY		
1a. Plank	2	45–60 seconds
1b. Side plank	1	30–45 seconds (each side)
STRENGTH: PRIMARY EXERCISES		
2. Squat	4	6
3a. Bench press	4	6
3b. Dumbbell three-point dead-start row	4	6 (each side)
STRENGTH: COMPLEMENTARY EXERCISES		
4a. Glute bridge	2	10–12
4b. Pike or inverted pushup	2	12–15
4c. Pulldown	2	12–15

What Do Those Numbers and Letters Mean?

When there's a number and a letter, you do those exercises as a circuit, or as alternating sets. So with the core exercises, you do the plank (1a) for as long as you can hold it; then you do the side plank (1b), working both sides; then you do the plank again.

With primary strength exercises, take as much rest as you need between each set of each exercise. So if you're alternating bench presses and rows, you'll do the first set of bench presses, rest, do the first set of rows, rest, and continue like that. For complementary and accessory exercises, you decide how much or how little rest you want to take. I typically do those exercises with no rest in between anything, except the time it takes to record a set in my training log.

When you see a number by itself, it means you do all the sets of that exercise with whatever amount of rest you need in between, then move on to the next exercise.

You don't *have* to alternate the lettered exercises. Sometimes the gym is too busy to allow it. Sometimes it's too inconvenient. And sometimes you just don't like to train that way. Remember, it's *your* workout.

WORKOUT 2

EXERCISE	SETS	REPS
CORE TRAINING: DYNAMIC STABILITY		
1. Dead bug	2	10–12 (each leg)
STRENGTH: PRIMARY EXERCISES		
2. Deadlift	3	8–10
3a. Shoulder press	3	8–10
3b. Chinup/pullup/inverted row*	3	8–10
STRENGTH: COMPLEMENTARY EXERCISES		
4a. Lunge	2	10–12 (each leg)
4b. Pushup	2	15
4c. Cable row*	2	15

*Use different grips. If you use an overhand grip for inverted rows, for example, use an underhand grip for cable rows.

WORKOUT 3

EXERCISE	SETS	REPS
CORE TRAINING: STRENGTH AND HYPERTROPHY		
1. McGill curlup	2	6–8 (each side)
STRENGTH: PRIMARY/COMPLEMENTARY EXERCISES		
2. Kettlebell swing	2–3	10–12
3a. T pushup	3	Max
3b. Inverted row	3	Max
STRENGTH: COMPLEMENTARY/ACCESSORY EXERCISES		
4. Farmer's walk	2–3	30 steps or 30 seconds
5a. Biceps curl	3	10–12
5b. Triceps extension	3	10–12

"Max" means "to momentary muscular exhaustion"—that is, the last full-range-of-motion repetition you can do with proper form. That's slightly different than "to failure," which suggests you keep going even after your form breaks down and you're reduced to doing partial reps.

PHASE TWO

WORKOUT 1

EXERCISE	SETS	REPS
CORE TRAINING: STABILITY		
1. Long-lever plank	2	30–60 seconds
STRENGTH: PRIMARY EXERCISES		
2. Sumo deadlift	4	6-6-4-4
3a. Shoulder press	3	8
3b. Chinup/pullup/lat pulldown	3	8
STRENGTH: COMPLEMENTARY EXERCISES		
4a. Cable single-arm row	2	12 (each side)
4b. Cable chest press	2	12 (each side)
5. Waiter's walk	2	30 steps or 30 seconds (each side)

Why 6-6-4-4?

In Phase One, the goal was to work with heavier weights from week to week. Here, on one or two exercises per workout, you want to use more weight on each set. So for the sumo deadlifts, you probably want to start with a warmup set. Then, on the first set of 6 reps, choose a weight you could probably lift for about 8 reps. On the next set of 6, use a heavier weight, one that you could probably lift for just 7 reps. Then go heavier for the next set: Although it calls for 4 reps, you want a weight you think you could lift 6 times. For the final set of 4, choose a weight you think you could lift 5 times.

In each subsequent week, you want to increase the weights you use for each set. So you don't want to be too aggressive or ambitious with your first-week choices.

WORKOUT 2

EXERCISE	SETS	REPS
CORE TRAINING: DYNAMIC STABILITY		
1. Pallof press	2	8–10 (each side)
STRENGTH: PRIMARY EXERCISES		
2a. Bench press	4	6-6-4-4
2b. Dumbbell or barbell row	4	6-6-4-4
3. Squat	3	8
STRENGTH: COMPLEMENTARY EXERCISES		
4a. Lunge	2	10–12 (each leg)
4b. Pike pushup	2	15
4c. Pulldown	2	15

WORKOUT 3

EXERCISE	SETS	REPS
CORE TRAINING: STRENGTH AND HYPERTROPHY		
1. Half Turkish getup	2–3	3–5 (each side)
STRENGTH: PRIMARY/COMPLEMENTARY EXERCISES		
2. Glute bridge	2–3	8–10
3a. Dumbbell incline single-arm bench press	2	10–12 (each arm)
3b. Single-arm half-kneeling lat pulldown	2	10–12 (each arm)
STRENGTH: COMPLEMENTARY/ACCESSORY EXERCISES		
4. Suitcase carry	2–3	30 steps or 30 seconds (each side)
5a. Biceps curl	3	10–12
5b. Triceps extension	3	10–12

PHASE THREE

These workouts employ a technique called *wave loading*. For squats and deadlifts, you'll do sets of 8, 5, 3, and 10 reps; for pushes and pulls, you'll do sets of 8, 5, 3, 10, and 12. Let's look at squats as an example of how to do this. We'll assume you're an experienced lifter whose 1-rep max is about 200 pounds.

Warmup. The first set calls for 8 reps, but you want to use a heavy weight here, one you think you could lift 10 times in an all-out set. That would be about 75 percent of your 1-rep max, which in this example would be 150 pounds. Before you tackle that set, you want to do at least 1 warmup set. To keep it simple and efficient, you'd probably use 95 pounds: the Olympic bar with a 25-pound plate on each side.

Escalating loads. The first 3 sets call for 8, 5, and 3 reps, with heavier weights on each. You know you're going to use 150 pounds for 8 reps on the first set (although you may round it down to 145 or up to 155, just so you don't have to mess with $2\frac{1}{2}$-pound plates).

For your heaviest set, 3 reps, you want to use about 90 percent of your max, which is a weight you could lift at most four times. In this case, that's 180 pounds.

The set in between calls for 5 reps. For that, you want to split the difference, which in this example would be 165 pounds.

It works best when you figure all this out in advance, including the amount you plan to use for your warmup set(s).

Back-off sets. These sets are what make pyramids fun. For the set of 10, I like to use the same weight I started with, the weight I used for 8 reps. It'll feel light at first, but believe me, that will change by the end of the set.

On pushes and pulls, you'll do a second back-off set, this one 12 reps. You want to drop the weight by about 20 percent. Again, it'll feel light at first, until it doesn't.

You'll face an interesting challenge when you reach the chinup/pullup/lat pulldown. I don't imagine many of you will be able to do chinups or pullups for all 5 sets. So here are some guidelines.

If you can do at least 1 set of 9 or 10 chinups or pullups: Do 8 with your body weight for the first set. Do weighted chinups or pullups for the sets of 5 and 3 reps. Then do lat pulldowns for the sets of 10 and 12. Try to use more weight each week.

If you can do 5 to 8 chinups or pullups: Do lat pulldowns for the set of 8. Do 5 chinups or pullups with your body weight. Add a light weight for the set of 3, and then do the two back-off sets with lat pulldowns. Try to use more weight each week for the set of 3; it's a major win if you can use a weight for the set of 5 as well.

If you can do fewer than 5 chinups or pullups: Do lat pulldowns for the sets of 8 and 5 reps. Do as many chinups or pullups as you can for the middle set, even if it's more than three. If you can only do one, do that three times. If you can't do one, boost yourself up to the top position (chest even with the bar), and lower yourself as slowly as possible. Do that 3 times.

First and Second 3 Weeks

Phase Three is designed to go 6 weeks. That way you get to use pyramids for all the primary exercises, doing each one 3 weeks at a time.

WORKOUT 1: FIRST 3 WEEKS

EXERCISE	SETS	REPS
CORE TRAINING: STABILITY		
1. Contralateral core lift	2	30 seconds
STRENGTH: PRIMARY EXERCISES		
2. Squat	4	8-5-3-10
3a. Bench press	3	8
3b. Dumbbell or barbell row	3	8
STRENGTH: COMPLEMENTARY EXERCISES		
4a. Lat pulldown	2	12
4b. Dumbbell or kettlebell single-arm shoulder press	2	12 (each side)
5. Overhead carry*	2	30 steps or 30 seconds

*Yes, it's incredibly fatiguing to do overhead carries right after pulldowns and shoulder presses—also kind of fun! Although you may want to use a different f-word to describe it.

WORKOUT 1: SECOND 3 WEEKS

EXERCISE	SETS	REPS
CORE TRAINING: STABILITY		
1. Choose your own	2	30 seconds
STRENGTH: PRIMARY EXERCISES		
2a. Bench press	5	8-5-3-10-12
2b. Dumbbell or barbell row	5	8-5-3-10-12
3. Squat	3	8
STRENGTH: COMPLEMENTARY EXERCISES		
4a. Lat pulldown	2	12
4b. Dumbbell or kettlebell single-arm shoulder press	2	12 (each side)
5. Overhead carry	2	30 steps or 30 seconds

WORKOUT 2: FIRST 3 WEEKS

EXERCISE	SETS	REPS
CORE TRAINING: DYNAMIC STABILITY		
1a. Rollout	2	8–10
1b. Swiss ball Jackknife	2	8–10
STRENGTH: PRIMARY EXERCISES		
2a. Shoulder press	5	8-5-3-10-12
2b. Chinup/pullup/lat pulldown	5	8-5-3-10-12
3. Deadlift	3	8
STRENGTH: COMPLEMENTARY EXERCISES		
4a. Lunge	2	10–12 (each leg)
4b. Pushup	2	15–20
4c. Cable row	2	15

WORKOUT 2: SECOND 3 WEEKS

EXERCISE	SETS	REPS
CORE TRAINING: DYNAMIC STABILITY		
1a. Choose your own	2	8–10
1b. Choose your own	2	8–10
STRENGTH: PRIMARY EXERCISES		
2. Deadlift	4	8-5-3-10
3a. Chinup/pullup/lat pulldown	3	8
3b. Shoulder press	3	8
STRENGTH: COMPLEMENTARY EXERCISES		
4a. Lunge	2	10–12 (each leg)
4b. Pushup	2	15–20
4c. Cable row	2	15

WORKOUT 3*

EXERCISE	SETS	REPS
CORE TRAINING: STRENGTH AND HYPERTROPHY		
1. Partial dragon flag	2 or 3	3–5
STRENGTH: PRIMARY/COMPLEMENTARY EXERCISES		
2. Stepup	2 or 3	10–12 (each side)
3a. Dumbbell incline crush press	3	10
3b. Inverted row (feet elevated)	3	10
STRENGTH: COMPLEMENTARY/ACCESSORY EXERCISES		
4. Farmer's walk	2 or 3	30 steps or 30 seconds
5a. Biceps curl	3	10–12
5b. Triceps extension	3	10–12

*Do the same program all 6 weeks.

CHAPTER 13:

PRIMARY EXERCISES

TRAINING WOULD BE BLESSEDLY SIMPLE and straightforward if all of us could do the exact same exercises with the exact same form and the exact same expectation of maximal results with minimal risk. Human physiology sneers at such utopian dreams. Consider my own tale of woe.

I started lifting when I was 13, but I didn't learn to squat and deadlift until my late thirties. That was a mistake of omission, which of course I had plenty of time to rectify. Alas, my first squats and deads coincided with a mistake of commission: I started playing pickup basketball with co-workers around that same time. Nothing wrong with that—except we played on concrete and asphalt, and it wasn't long before I composted my knee cartilage.

I still managed to develop decent strength for a late starter. I got a double-body-weight deadlift in my midforties, and I'm pretty sure my best squat was about one and two-thirds my weight at the time. But I hurt my knee trying to exceed that squat PR, and I've never gotten close to it since. In fact, I can't remember the last time I even tried to squat with a barbell on my back. I got along fine with front squats for a few years, but then some abdominal injuries made those problematic as well.

Today I use weights that are heavy by regular-guy-in-a-typical-health-club standards, while genuinely strong guys might not even warm up with my max. You may be one of them. But here's something I learned in the process of getting older, training around injuries, and accommodating the indignities of flawed physiology: *It absolutely doesn't matter* how much weight you lift. Or which exercises you can or can't do.

That's why in Chapter 12 you'll see so many places where I tell you to do a squat or deadlift, or a bench or shoulder press, or a lunge or pulldown variation, but don't tell you which one. The best one for you is the one you can do with the best form, least discomfort, and heaviest load within the designated range of sets and reps.

What matters are how hard and consistently you train, what capacities you develop, and the degree to which those capacities exceed your current levels. Do that and you *will* get stronger, even if you never get genuinely strong. You *will* develop more muscle, even if you never reach the point where, if you're a suspect in a crime, eyewitnesses describe you to police as "muscular." ("Well, officer, it was dark, but I could tell he was muscular because he had the classic shoulder-to-waist ratio of 1.6. Also because he stopped to show me his front double biceps pose.") And if your training coincides with Alan's diet plan, you *will* get leaner, even if no one ever mistakes you for a fitness model.

Do those things, and you're better off than not just the majority of the population, who don't exercise at all, but also the majority of people who exercise without much to show for it.

Squat Exercises

"Squats can do more for total mass and body strength than probably all other lifts combined," strength coach Dan John wrote in an article for T-nation. com. "Doing them wrong can do more damage than probably all the other moves, too."

Here's how Dan describes the right way to do them.

1. Stand.

2. Spread your feet just a bit beyond shoulder-width apart, with your toes either pointed straight ahead or angled out slightly.

3. Extend your arms or clasp your hands in front of your chest.

4. Push your chest out. This automatically pulls your lats down, which will help keep your lower back and pelvis locked in the neutral position.

5. Push your buttocks back and descend into a squat.

6. Return to the starting position.

7. Repeat multiple times every day for the rest of your life.

That's how you groove the movement pattern. To build muscle with that movement pattern, you'll need to use one or more of the following variations. If you're experienced in all three squat variations, choose the one you feel is best for your goals. The exercise behind Door Number 3, the back squat, allows the heaviest loading, and thus the greatest overall strength and mass development. But don't underestimate the potential of the other two.

If you're not confident or experienced in any of them, I *beg* you to start with the goblet squat, and move up to the front squat only when you reach the exercise's natural limits—your lower-body strength exceeds the amount of weight you can hold against your chest, or you reach the end of your gym's dumbbell rack and the only way to use heavier weights is with a barbell.

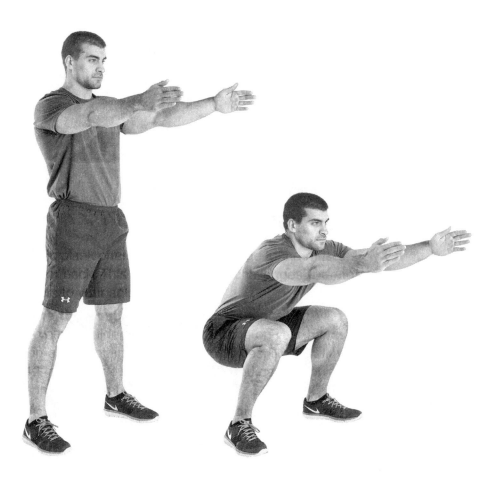

1. GOBLET SQUAT

Do not, under any circumstances, assume that this exercise isn't manly enough for you. If you've tried it and thought it was easy, try it again, this time with enough weight to make it hard.

Assume the position: Grab a dumbbell or kettlebell and hold it with both hands against your chest. Hold a dumbbell parallel to your torso, with your hands on either side of the top end. You can hold the kettlebell with your hands around the base or on the sides of the handle.

Work:

1. Push your hips back and lower yourself until the tops of your thighs are parallel to the floor, or a bit lower if you can.

2. Return to the starting position.

DUMBBELL GOBLET SQUAT   **KETTLEBELL GOBLET SQUAT**

BIG-BOY TIP:

You can do goblet squats with any amount of weight, as long as you can lift the weight into the starting position. For a heavier dumbbell, first set it upright on a box or bench. Squat down and grab the bell with the base of your palms under the top-end weight and your fingers spread out over the sides. Now stand, using your momentum to lift the weight up to your chest. Set your feet and you're ready to go.

2. FRONT SQUAT

Assume the position:

1. Place a barbell in the squat rack so it's just below shoulder height.

2. Take a shoulder-width, overhand grip, then rotate your arms under the bar until your elbows point straight out, your upper arms are parallel to the floor, and the bar rests on your palms.

3. As you lift the bar off the supports, let it roll back so it rests behind the groove at the base of your front deltoids. As long as you keep your elbows up, the bar will stay locked in that position.

4. Step back from the rack and set your feet as described on page 212.

Work:

1. Push your hips back and lower yourself until the tops of your thighs are parallel to the floor, or a bit lower if you can.

2. Return to the starting position.

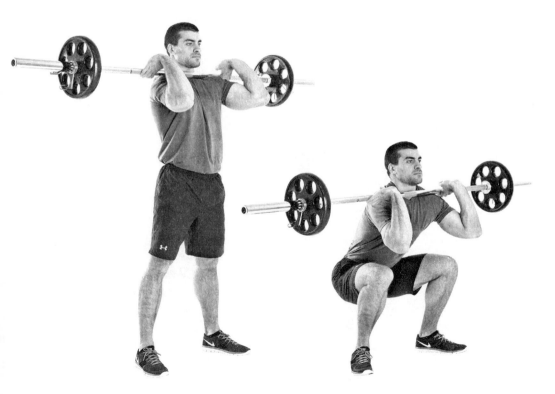

3. BACK SQUAT

Purists don't like using any modifier before the word "squat." To them, a squat is done with a barbell on the back. Everything else requires an adjective. Me, I'm a different kind of purist. I think "squat" is a movement pattern, and "back squat" is the most advanced application of that movement pattern. But their purists can beat up our purists, so take my opinion in the spirit of humility in which it's intended.

Assume the position:

1. Place a barbell in the squat rack so it's just below shoulder height.

2. Grab the bar with your hands outside shoulder width.

3. Duck under the bar and squeeze your shoulders together, creating a platform for the bar with your upper traps.

4. Lift the bar, step back from the rack, and set your feet as described on page 212.

Work:

1. Push your hips back and descend until the tops of your thighs are parallel to the floor.

2. Return to the starting position.

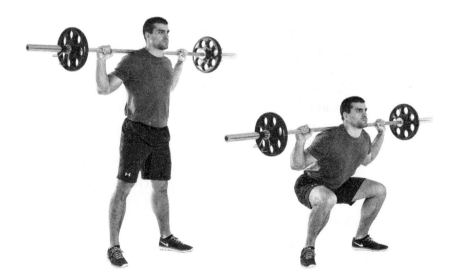

Deadlift Exercises

Mike Boyle, strength coach for the Boston Red Sox and a former powerlifter, has a great quote about the deadlift: "You can't deadlift heavy and well." If you don't believe it, he wrote, go to a powerlifting meet and watch what happens when the barbell hits the floor. "It makes you cringe to watch."

So forget how much weight you can pull off the floor. Unless you're a competitive lifter, who cares? The key to using the lift successfully is to engage the right muscles in the right movement pattern, and then get as strong as you can without compromising that form.

If you've never deadlifted before, I recommend starting with option 1, the conventional style. The other two variations—sumo and hex-bar deadlifts—might ultimately be a better fit for your body. But you should at least try the classic technique first. I used it exclusively for many years, and got decently strong without any problems. It became uncomfortable for me only after a series of injuries unrelated to deadlifting. (As far as I know; injury origins aren't always apparent.)

I switched to option 2, the sumo deadlift, during a group workout at a fitness conference. All the men and several women in the group I was lifting with were stronger than I was. I used the sumo style because they did. Even though I'd never trained with it, I kept up with them longer than I thought I could, pulling weights I hadn't touched in recent memory. Now I use sumo most of the time.

Option 3, the hex-bar deadlift, is also a good option for many lifters. Some coaches consider it a squat–deadlift hybrid, since you use your quadriceps more than you would in the other styles. My recommendation is to try the conventional and sumo deadlifts before moving on to the hex bar. (This assumes your gym has one, or that you can afford to buy one for a home gym.)

If you have experience with all three, pick the one that works best for you. You can use one style for all three phases of the program, or use a different one each time. Yes, what you have here is something stated most convincingly by Mel Gibson in *Braveheart*: "Freedom!" (Extra points if you can explain how his character managed to shout this after having his intestines removed with an iron hook.)

Before You Get Started

All these deadlift descriptions assume you can start with a 45-pound weight plate on each side of the Olympic bar. Counting the 45-pound bar, that's 135 pounds, and it puts the bar about 8 inches off the floor. But if you can't yet train with 135 pounds, you have to make some adjustments. Starting with lighter weights means the bar will sit a couple inches lower. You have to bend farther to lift it, which increases the risk to your lower back.

You have a couple options.

1. If your gym has bumper plates—lighter plates that are 17 inches in diameter, the same size as the 45s—use those.

2. No bumper plates? You can set the bar on a pair of low boxes or steps, or on the safety bars of a squat rack.

3. No matter your strength or experience, you want to start with your feet as close to the ground as possible. That means wearing the flattest shoes you can find—or lifting without shoes, if you train at home or at a gym where you can get away with it.

1. CONVENTIONAL DEADLIFT

People who are really, really strong in the conventional style tend to have spinal erectors—the parallel bands of muscle in the lower and middle back—that look like braunschweiger rolls. So, naturally, I've always assumed that conventional deadlifts use those muscles more than the other techniques. But when researchers look at muscle and joint actions across the various deadlift styles, that's not what jumps out. Conventional deadlifts involve a lot more action at the hip joints—that is, more work for the glutes and hamstrings—and also more total energy expenditure, since it takes longer to complete each repetition. They also use the calves more and the quads less.

Assume the position:

1. Set the loaded barbell on the floor.

2. Put your shins up against the bar, with your feet shoulder-width apart and your toes straight ahead or angled out slightly.

3. Bend over and grab the bar with your hands just outside your legs.

4. Push your hips back.

5. Now comes absolutely the most important part: Grab the bar like the future of human civilization depends on it. A hard grip naturally tightens the rest of your body.

6. As you strangle the bar (seriously, try to inflict pain on it), push your chest up and pull your shoulders down, which will naturally brace your core and fix your lower back in its natural arch.

Work:

1. Pull the weight off the floor, bringing it straight up along your shins.

2. As the bar passes your knees, thrust your hips forward.

3. Finish the lift by squeezing your glutes and shoulder blades.

4. Push your hips back and lower the bar to the floor under control.

5. Reset your grip and tighten your body for the next lift.

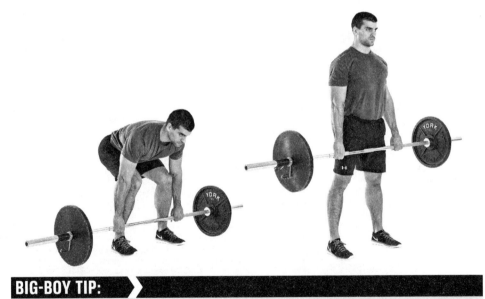

BIG-BOY TIP:

I used to focus my eyes straight ahead when deadlifting, which means my neck was slightly hyperextended, rather than aligned with my back and pelvis. In recent years I've followed Mark Rippetoe's advice to set my gaze to a spot that would be about 12 to 15 feet in front of me. I don't know if it makes me stronger, but it feels like my form is more consistent from one rep to the next.

2. SUMO DEADLIFT

With the wide stance, you're using more of your lower-body muscles, including the quads and the adductors (inner thigh muscles). You also start in a more upright position and take less time to complete each rep, so there's a bit less of a challenge to your lower back.

Assume the position:

1. Step up to the barbell with a double-shoulder-width stance and toes pointed out about 45 degrees.

2. Bend over and grab the bar with your arms inside your legs and about shoulder-width apart.

3. Push your hips back, tighten your grip, lift your chest, and pull your shoulders down.

Work:

1. Pull the bar off the floor, thrusting your hips forward as the bar passes your knees.

2. Squeeze your glutes and shoulder blades to finish the lift.

3. Lower the weight under control, and reset for the next rep.

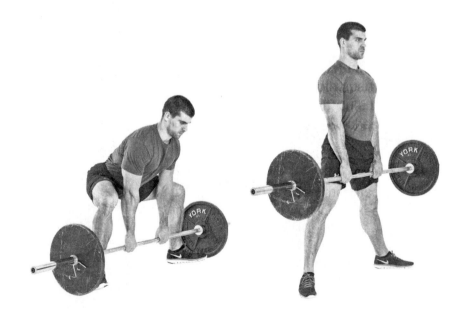

3. HEX-BAR DEADLIFT

Before you start, you need to know your equipment. Most hex bars in gyms today have two sets of handles. The lower handles will be the usual 8 inches above the floor when lifting 45-pound plates. The second set is several inches higher, which cuts the range of motion and allows you to lift heavier weights. Unlike Olympic barbells, which always weigh 45 pounds (technically, they're 44 pounds/20 kilograms, but we round it up to 45 to keep the math simple), there's no standard weight for a hex bar. It might be 45 pounds, or 50, or 55. It also could be less. It only matters if you're the rare #humblebrag douche who likes to tweet his massive hex-bar-deadlift numbers.

One more note: When I use the low handles on the hex bar, it feels like I'm lifting from a much lower position than the conventional deadlift. I feel a dull strain in my back and a sharp strain in my knees. The lift feels natural only with the high handles.

Assume the position:

1. Load the bar and stand in the middle with your feet shoulder-width apart and toes pointed forward.

2. Squat down and grab the handles.

(continued)

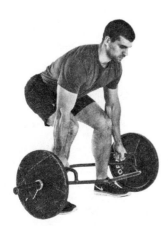

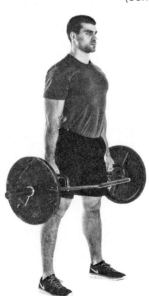

3. As with any other deadlift, push your hips back, tighten your grip, lift your chest, and pull your shoulders down.

Work:

1. Pull the weight straight up off the floor.

2. Squeeze your glutes and shoulder blades to finish the lift.

3. Lower the weight under control, and reset for the next rep.

BIG-BOY TIP:

One study of experienced powerlifters showed they could use 8 percent more weight with the hex bar than with conventional deadlifts. The disparity might be even greater with less experienced lifters. My guess is that a lot of gym rats and noncompetitive lifters can use heavier weights with the hex bar than with any other free-weight exercise. Strength coach Jason Ferruggia suggests the increased strength comes with increased risk. A straight bar acts as a natural restraint for your hips, since your legs are in contact with it at the start and finish of each rep. With a trap bar, your hips are moving freely. The heavier the weight, the more risk there is for an errant movement.

Push Exercises

Most of the pushing movements we do in daily life are no more strenuous than opening a door. When we lift something overhead, it's rarely anything heavy. *How* we do it doesn't matter much. But what happens when you need to push something really big and heavy, like a car that's stuck in the mud?

Here's what you wouldn't do: You wouldn't sit down in the mud with your chest against the rear bumper and try to move it by straightening your arms. You instinctively understand the car won't go anywhere unless you put your entire body into the task.

So you stand up, lean forward with your shoulders against the car, and drive your legs with all the force you can muster. While your lower-body muscles strain against the load, your core tightens to protect your lower back. You flex your upper-back muscles to create a platform behind your shoulders. Only then—as the final part of a complex, total-body movement—do you try to straighten your arms.

Like I said, you do all that without being told. I can't think of a single situation in which you'd try to push a heavy object without throwing everything you have into the task. But when we get to the weight room, we immediately disregard natural, instinctive movement principles in favor of exercises that attempt to isolate muscle groups.

The bench press is the best example. Strength coaches sometimes refer to it as a "horizontal" press, even though the weight moves vertically. The goal of the nomenclature, I suppose, is to distinguish it from an overhead press, which is obviously vertical. But it serves another purpose: If you were on your feet, literally pushing a weight horizontally, you'd treat it as a total-body movement. (The standing cable chest press, which you'll find in the next chapter, is a perfect example.) Competitive lifters understand this; if you ever watch a powerlifting competition, you'll see how important the lower body is to the force they generate.

CHEST PRESS 1: DUMBBELL BENCH PRESS

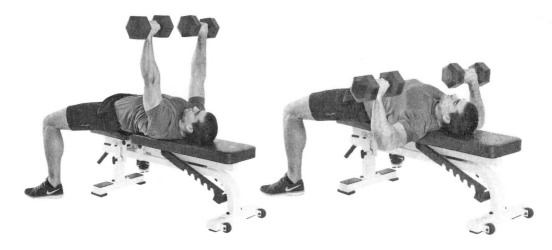

Assume the position:

1. Grab a pair of dumbbells and lie on your back on a flat bench. (You can also set the bench at an incline between 30 and 45 degrees, either for variety or to alleviate shoulder discomfort.)

2. Hold the weights straight up over your shoulders. Most of us do this with our palms out, but some prefer to turn the palms in. Whatever feels best for your shoulders is fine; I don't think your pecs will know the difference.

3. Spread your knees wide apart, with your feet on the floor. For the heaviest weights, twist the balls of your feet outward, like you're trying to screw them into the floor.

4. Arch your back; only your buttocks, upper back, and the back of your head should rest on the bench.

Work:

1. Lower the weights to the outside edges of your shoulders. If you have long arms, you can stop when your upper arms are even with the bench.

2. Push the weights straight up from your shoulders and repeat.

CHEST PRESS 2: DUMBBELL INCLINE SINGLE-ARM BENCH PRESS

This variation, designated for Phase Two, Workout 3, challenges your core, and also helps you build balanced strength on both sides of your torso.

Assume the position:

1. Set the bench to a 45-degree angle.

2. Grab a single dumbbell and lie on your back on the bench, holding the weight at the edge of your shoulder. You can do whatever you want with your nonworking arm. (I prefer to rest mine on my stomach.)

3. Spread your knees and set your feet flat on the floor.

Work:

1. Push the weight straight up toward the ceiling.

2. Lower the weight to the starting position and repeat. After completing all reps, repeat with the opposite arm.

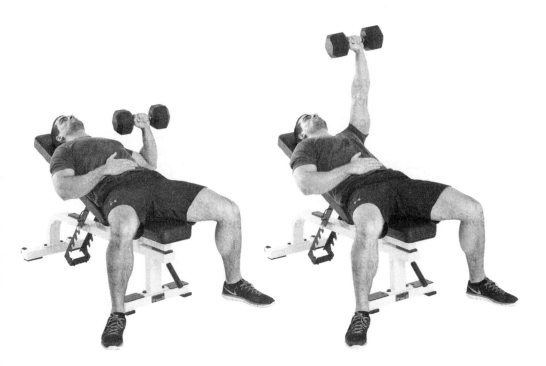

CHEST PRESS 3: DUMBBELL INCLINE CRUSH PRESS

When you get to this variation in Phase Three, Workout 3, you may find it to be the best triceps exercise in the program. It's also a different kind of stimulation for your chest and core.

Assume the position:

1. Set the bench to an incline of 30 to 45 degrees.

2. Grab a pair of dumbbells and lie on your back on the bench, holding the weights in front of your chest with your palms facing each other and the sides of the dumbbells touching.

Work:

1. As you press the weights straight up toward the ceiling, crush them together. The goal is to lift them as if they're a single object.

2. Pause, feel the squeeze in your chest and core, lower the weights, and repeat.

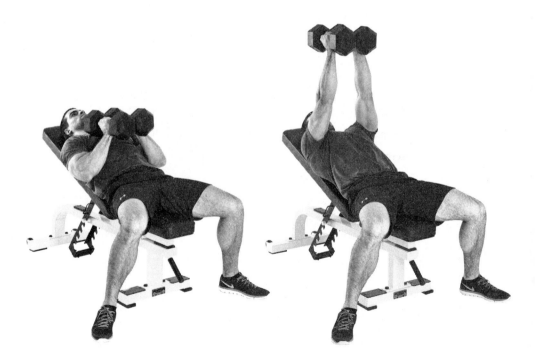

CHEST PRESS 4: BARBELL BENCH PRESS

This is one of just a handful of exercises in this book that I don't do. I come by my aversion to it honestly. I worked as hard as I could to build strength and skill with the barbell, but ultimately my sore shoulder got the final vote. I'm also lucky enough to train at a gym with dumbbells that go beyond my current strength.

But some of you will need to use the barbell bench press. If you work out at home, you don't have the option of buying full sets of heavy dumbbells in 5-pound increments. Even if you lift in a gym, there are limits. A pair of 100-pound-plus dumbbells costs hundreds of dollars. Then the gym owners have to spend hundreds more on a rack specially engineered for those superheavy weights.

If you have any aspiration to compete in powerlifting, you obviously need to master the barbell press. The same probably applies to any strength and power athlete. For maximal upper-body strength development, there's really no other option.

For everyone else, I encourage you to stick with dumbbells as long as you can. Since each arm moves independently, they're safer for your shoulders. They also add *work* to your workouts. In a gym, the heaviest weights are typically on the bottom row of the dumbbell rack, and it takes some effort to lift them out and put them back. The steps from the rack to your bench are the equivalent of heavy carries, a key complementary exercise in the program. It all adds up, and shouldn't be underestimated. But for those who need (or just want) to use the barbell, here's how to do it.

Assume the position:

1. Load the barbell and lie on your back on a flat or incline bench.

2. Spread your knees and set your feet on the floor.

3. Grab the bar with your hands about one and a half times wider than shoulder width.

4. Lift the bar off the supports. (For the heaviest lifts, get a spotter to hand it off to you.)

5. Tighten everything up, from your feet to your core (keep your back arched) to your upper back (pull your shoulder blades together) to your hands (as with the deadlift, a tight grip helps tighten everything).

Work:

1. Flex your lats and *pull the bar down* to your lower chest, keeping your elbows in close to your torso.

2. Touch the bar to your chest and push the bar back up to the starting position.

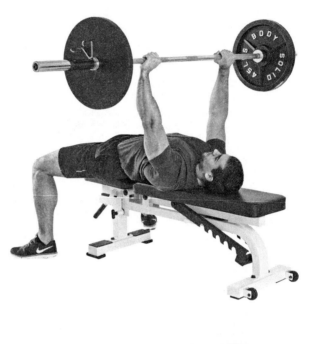

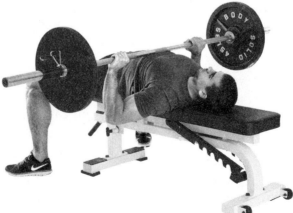

OVERHEAD PRESS 1: DUMBBELL SHOULDER PRESS

This may be the only overhead press some of you need. It should work your shoulders, upper traps, and triceps as well as any exercise can. It's easier on your shoulders than the barbell version. And if you train in a gym, you aren't likely to outgrow the available selection of dumbbells. In a lifetime of workouts I don't think I've ever used more than 60 pounds in each hand.

Assume the position:

1. Grab a pair of dumbbells and stand holding them at the sides of your shoulders. You can turn your palms out or in toward each other; many find the latter feels more comfortable. It shouldn't make any major difference to your muscles.

2. Set your feet shoulder-width apart, with your toes pointed forward.

Work:

1. Push the weights straight up over your shoulders.

2. Lower them and repeat.

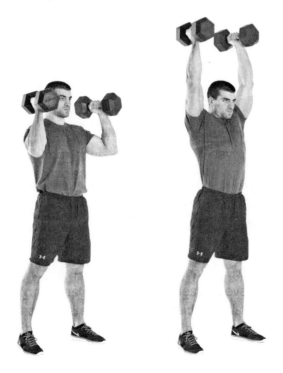

OVERHEAD PRESS 2: BARBELL SHOULDER PRESS

When my brother and I started working out in our basement, circa 1970, this was probably the first exercise we attempted. We didn't have a bench, so to us, the military press, as it was commonly known, was the only press that mattered. It was even an Olympic lift from 1928 to 1972, along with the snatch and clean and jerk. The latter two exercises were considered "quick lifts," while the press was thought to be a test of pure strength. The press was abandoned in the Olympics because it was difficult to judge. What started as a slow, strict lift—heels together, eyes forward—had become fast and loose, with lifters leaning back to use their chest muscles along with their shoulders and arms.

The end of Olympic pressing severed the last connection between the three strength sports—powerlifting, bodybuilding, and Olympic weightlifting. Bodybuilders still did the three powerlifts, but with Olympic lifting already in steep decline, the military press became an afterthought. All bragging rights went to the bench press, while the shoulder press turned into a pure muscle-building tool. Bodybuilders no longer lifted the bar from the floor to their shoulders. The seated version became more popular than the standing press, typically with the back braced against an upright pad, and it was often performed behind the neck.

I don't want to say the standing barbell press is due for a renaissance, but I do think it's worth a try if you have no recent history of shoulder or back problems. When I started using it again, I was surprised by how natural it felt. It's still hard, in that it feels like a total-body challenge. But I don't experience any discomfort at all, despite having had shoulder problems off and on since high school.

Assume the position:

1. Set the bar in the supports of a squat rack just below shoulder height. (You can start with it on the floor if you know how to do a clean.)

2. Grab the bar with your hands just outside shoulder width; don't hesitate to go wider if it's more comfortable and you feel stronger.

3. Slide your hands under the bar until your arms are in front of your torso and your forearms are more or less perpendicular to the floor.

4. Lift the bar off the supports and step back, setting your feet about hip-width apart.

5. Rest the bar at the base of your throat, right below your chin, and look straight ahead or slightly up toward the ceiling.

Work:

1. Push the bar straight up, leaning your head back just enough to avoid smashing your chin or nose.

2. Bring your head back to alignment as you push the weight to lockout overhead.

3. Pause, then lean your head back again, lower the bar to the base of your throat, and repeat.

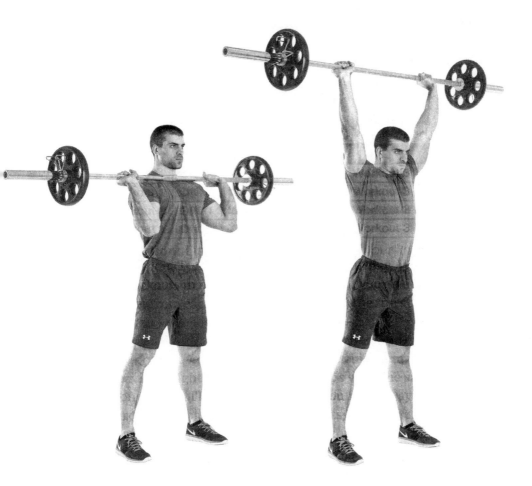

This one is on me: Most of the time, when you see a barbell shoulder press in a fitness magazine or workout book, the model holds the bar in front of his shoulders, with his upper arms aligned with his torso and his elbows pointing toward the floor. From there he could lift and lower the bar without having to move his head out of the way. I don't pretend to have a perfect understanding of the biomechanics, but it seems like that's a riskier position for the shoulders. Your spine provides the base of support when you lift straight over your head, but when the weight is out in front of your torso, that support is reduced to the tendons and ligaments in the shoulder joints. My advice, which applies to pretty much any exercise you're tempted to try: If the form you see in photos or videos doesn't feel right to you, you can either move on to another exercise—there's no shortage of choices, for any movement pattern— or find a better example.

Pull Exercises

Horizontal pulling exercises are blessedly simple compared with horizontal pushes. For one thing, they're actually horizontal the way we do them most of the time, with cable machines. For another, the exercises we call rows actually look like rowing—the thing you'd do if you were trying to get a boat from one side of a lake to the other.

Vertical pulls are similarly easy to comprehend. You don't need a degree in physiology to understand that a lat pulldown works the lats. (Not that anyone's confused about what a shoulder press works.)

The biggest trick is finding a way to balance pushes and pulls throughout a program. What looks like an even-steven mix on paper is often unbalanced in terms of intensity. Technically, "intensity" refers to "intensity of load," defined as the percentage of your 1-rep maximum that you use on any given exercise. But most often we use it to mean "intensity of effort"—how hard we think we're working. Some exercises simply feel harder than others. Right at the top of the list are chinups and pullups. (Chinups use an underhand grip, pullups an overhand grip.) They feel much tougher than the lat pulldown, which is the closest equivalent if we're going strictly by geometry. But if we try to match exercises according to the total-body effort required, the inverted row is most similar to the chinup or pullup, even though your body is diagonal rather than vertical.

That's why the workout charts in the previous chapter will sometimes say this: "Chinup/pullup/inverted row." If you can do either chinups or pullups for the designated sets and reps, you choose which you want to do. If you can't do either, you'll do inverted rows. Other times the chart will say "Chinup/pullup/lat pulldown." Same instructions: Do chinups or pullups if you can, lat pulldowns if you can't.

Those who can't do chinups or pullups for 8 or more reps will sometimes end up doing inverted rows or lat pulldowns in consecutive workouts, using them as both primary and complementary exercises. Redundant? Not really. Both exercises, as you'll see, are versatile enough to give you fresh challenges each time.

INVERTED ROW

This may be the most perfect upper-body pulling exercise ever invented. You can adjust your body to make it easier or harder, which means virtually any healthy person can do some version of it. By changing your grip and the angle of pull you can work your back and arms in slightly different ways from one set to the next, or from workout to workout.

Assume the position:

1. Set a barbell on the supports of a squat rack so it's about hip height. You can go a little higher to make it easier when you want to get more reps, or lower to make it more challenging.

2. Get beneath the bar and grab it overhand, with your hands about one and a half times shoulder width.

3. Hang from the bar at arm's length, with your body straight and your weight resting on your heels.

Work:

1. Pull your chest up to the bar.

2. Pause, return to the starting position, and repeat.

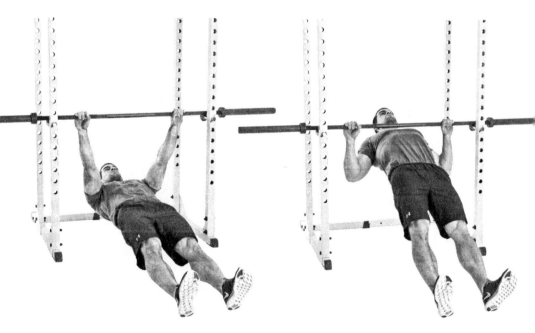

1. When you feel as if you're going to fall a few reps short of your target, bend your knees and bring your feet in a little. I can't think of another exercise that allows this big an adjustment in the middle of a set without shortening the range of motion.

2. You can widen your grip to put more emphasis on the upper-back muscles, including the rear delts and upper traps.

3. A narrower, underhand grip works the biceps and preferentially hits the middle-back muscles.

4. When you max out on these options, you can raise your feet on a box or bench to increase the challenge.

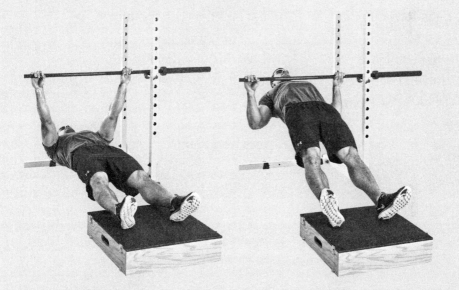

5. Another great option is the suspended row, using a suspension trainer like the TRX or Jungle Gym. It adds a stability challenge not only to your core, but also to the smaller muscles in your back and shoulders.

HORIZONTAL PULL 1: DUMBBELL THREE-POINT DEAD-START ROW

I've never liked the classic version of the bent-over row, with one hand and one knee resting on a bench. Your body is set up to allow so much torso rotation that you can lift heavy weights without fully engaging the upper-back muscles you're trying to work. The three-point row solves that problem by putting both feet on the floor. It's a more solid platform for lifting a heavy weight, and it helps keep your shoulders and hips square to the floor.

Assume the position:

1. Set a dumbbell on the floor next to a bench or sturdy box.

2. Stand facing the bench, your toes about 18 to 24 inches from it, and set your feet shoulder-width apart, or a little wider.

3. Lean forward at the hips and set one hand on the bench.

4. Reach down with your other hand and grab the dumbbell with your palm facing in and your hand directly below your shoulder.

5. Tighten everything, from your feet through your hands. It should feel a bit like the start of a deadlift.

Work:

1. Pull the weight to the side of your abdomen.

2. Lower the weight to the floor, reset your grip and your stance, and repeat. Do all the reps, then switch arms and repeat the set.

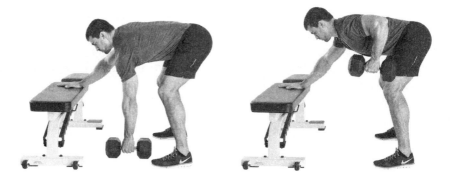

HORIZONTAL PULL 2: BARBELL ROW

Back in the day, this was a default exercise for bodybuilders. I tried it off and on, but I typically felt it more in my lower back than in the muscles I was trying to target. Yet again, the answer was to start each rep with the weight on the floor. That change also makes it more technically complex. You don't just set up once and grind out your reps. You reset your body for every single repetition. It's a great exercise for the most advanced and confident lifters, but one I don't recommend using for more than one phase of the program. Most important: Never do barbell rows and deadlifts in the same workout. The result would be an unacceptable amount of lower-back fatigue.

Assume the position:

1. You want the bar to start at the same height as in a deadlift. If you can't use 135 pounds, you'll need to use bumper plates. No bumper plates? Start with the bar on a pair of low boxes or the safety bars of a squat rack.

2. Set up as you would for a conventional deadlift, with your feet about shoulder-width apart and hands outside your legs.

3. Tighten up everything, starting with your grip.

Work:

1. Pull the bar straight up to your lower abdomen.

2. Lower it to the floor.

3. Reset your body and repeat.

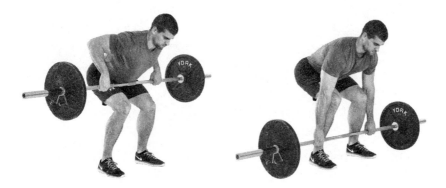

VERTICAL PULL 1: KNEELING LAT PULLDOWN

The original Universal multistation gym got one thing exactly right: The high-pulley station didn't have a seat. To use it for lat pulldowns, you had to kneel on the floor. I don't know who added the seat, or when, but I kind of wish they'd left it alone. When you sit on the machine, with your knees braced under the pad, you in effect cut your body in half. Normally, your glutes would combine with your lats to support your lower back. But when your hips are flexed 90 degrees, as they are when you sit, the glutes are stretched and get taken out of their role as a stabilizing force. Kneeling brings them back into the picture.

Assume the position:

1. Attach a long bar to the overhead pulley.

2. Grab the bar with a wide, overhand grip, and kneel on the floor, facing the weight stack.

Work:

1. Pull the bar to your upper chest, and at the same time push your chest out to meet the bar. That ensures the strongest contraction in your lats and traps.

2. Hold the contraction for a second, then return the bar to the starting position and repeat.

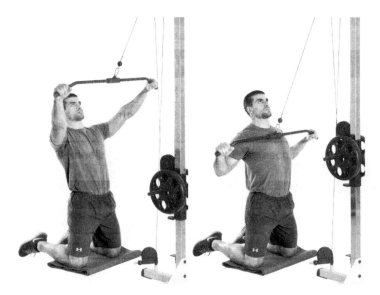

VERTICAL PULL 2: SINGLE-ARM HALF-KNEELING LAT PULLDOWN

This variation is designated for Phase Two, Workout 3.

Assume the position:

1. Attach a D-shaped handle to the high pulley.

2. Grab the handle with one hand, and step back just far enough to put tension on the cable when your arm is straight.

3. Kneel facing the cable machine, with your opposite knee forward.

4. Lift your chest, and tighten your core.

Work:

1. Pull the handle to the side of your chest, keeping your shoulders and hips square to the machine. (Your shoulders will rotate a bit, but try to minimize it.)

2. Pause for a second, then slowly straighten your arm to the starting position.

3. Do all your reps, then switch sides and repeat.

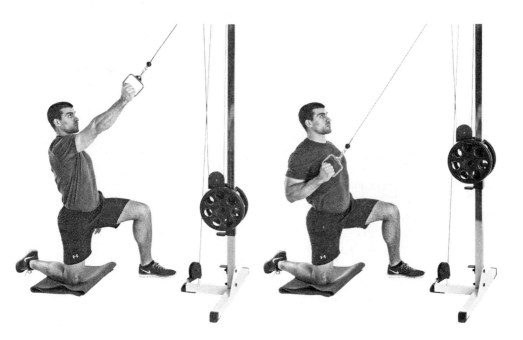

VERTICAL PULL 3: CHINUP OR PULLUP

Which you do is up to you. When I was in high school, we did an annual fitness test that included pullups. So when I worked out I would do double-digit sets as part of my warmup. I don't remember doing chinups until deep into adulthood, when pullups, for some mysterious reason, felt like getting stabbed in the shoulders.

I suspect most of us can do more chinups than pullups, and that those with lingering shoulder-joint issues will prefer them. If you can do both, feel free to alternate from program to program.

Just to keep it interesting, some gyms offer a neutral-grip option with a variety of widths. It's probably more of a chinup than pullup, but what you call it doesn't matter. Use it, don't use it. Totally up to you.

What matters for complete back and arm development is to use a variety of grips on your other pull exercises.

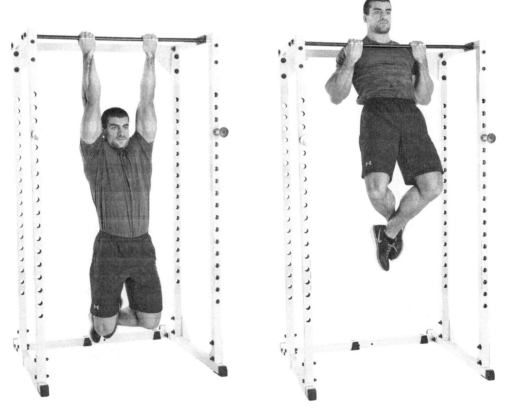

Assume the position: For chinups, use an underhand grip that's just inside shoulder width. For a pullup, use an overhand grip that's a little wider than your shoulders. Hang from the bar with straight arms. Most lifters prefer to bend their knees and cross their ankles behind them, but that's optional.

Work:

1. Pull your chest to the bar, or as close as you can get to it.

2. Pause, then lower yourself to the starting position and repeat.

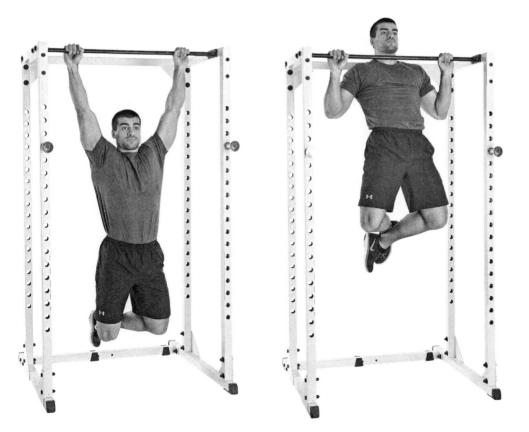

When you get to Phase Three, you'll do a variety of rep ranges, starting with 8, then 5, then 3, then back up again. The goal is to use more weight as you reduce reps, and less weight as you increase them. Since your body weight won't change from one set to the next, you have to add weight to your body. Many gyms have a dipping belt, which has a chain to hold a dumbbell or weight plate between your legs. You can also use a weighted vest or backpack.

CHAPTER 14:

COMPLEMENTARY AND ACCESSORY EXERCISES

MENTIONED IN CHAPTER 3 that there's no bright, clear line separating primary, complementary, and accessory exercises. Take the pushup. If 10 or 15 reps are a challenge, then the pushup can and probably should be a primary training exercise *for you*. It works your chest, shoulders, and triceps just the way you'd use them in a bench press. Same with a body-weight squat. It's a warmup exercise in the Lean Muscle Plan, but if you can't do 15 good reps, it becomes a serious lower-body training exercise.

The key difference among categories (as noted in Chapter 9) is how you do them. You do the primary exercises with the goal of getting stronger from one week to the next. Most of the time you'll finish a set knowing you could have gotten 1 or 2 more reps. You do the complementary and accessory exercises with the goal of pushing your muscles to what seems like their limit, at least for the moment.

Lunge Exercises

I'm agnostic when it comes to choosing the best exercises in this category. They all work the same muscles in more or less the same way. Let's look at the options.

HOW YOU MOVE

Split squat ("static" lunge): Stand with your feet together. Take one long step forward. For accounting purposes, the front leg is the working side. Drop until the top of the front thigh is parallel to the floor and the rear knee is close to the floor. Rise. That's 1 rep. Finish the set, then repeat with the opposite leg forward.

Reverse lunge: Just like in the warmups: Step back, drop, return to the starting position. You can do all the reps with one leg at a time, or alternate.

Forward lunge: Again, just like the warmups. Step forward, drop down, return to the starting position.

Walking lunge: You may find this easier on your knees than the forward lunge, since you're literally going forward on each rep, rather than stepping forward, stopping, and pushing back to the starting position. I consider it an advanced variation simply because the coordination is tricky, especially when you use one of the loading options described next.

HOW YOU LOAD IT

Dumbbells in both hands, arm's length: This is the variation you've seen in every fitness book and hundreds of workout articles—especially in women's magazines—since the beginning of time (depending, of course, on when time began for you). You can also use kettlebells.

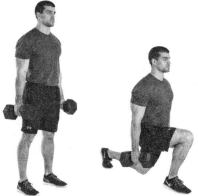

Dumbbell in one hand, shoulder-level: Hold the dumbbell on the same side as your working leg. So if you're doing a reverse lunge, for example, hold it in your left hand while stepping back with your right leg.

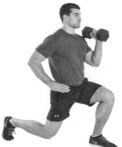

Dumbbell or kettlebell in one hand, overhead: This time, hold the weight in the hand opposite the working leg.

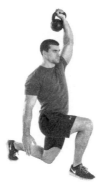

Weight(s) in front of you: You can have a lot of fun with these options:

▶ Single dumbbell, kettlebell, or weight plate in goblet position

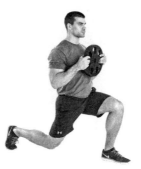

▶ Two kettlebells, rack position

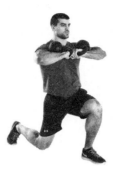

▶ Barbell, front-squat position

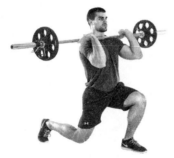

▶ Barbell or sandbag, Zercher-squat position (held in the crook of the arms in front of the abdomen)

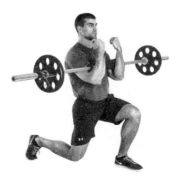

Weight behind you: You can hold a barbell or sandbag across the back of your shoulders, as you would in a squat.

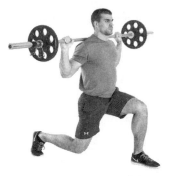

Weight(s) overhead: You can use a barbell, sandbag, weight plate, or two dumbbells or kettlebells.

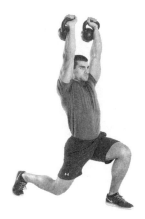

HOW YOU CHOOSE TO TORTURE YOURSELF

Rear-foot-elevated split squat: This has always been problematic for me. The goal of the exercise is to extend the range of motion of the standard split squat, which puts too much strain on my two most vulnerable areas: knees and lower abdomen. But for you it might be a great exercise. Set the toes of your rear foot on a low step (12 inches or lower), or rest your instep on a slightly higher step, box, or bench.

Try it with body weight only at first (hands behind your head in the prisoner grip), then advance to holding dumbbells at your sides, or a single weight in the goblet position as shown.

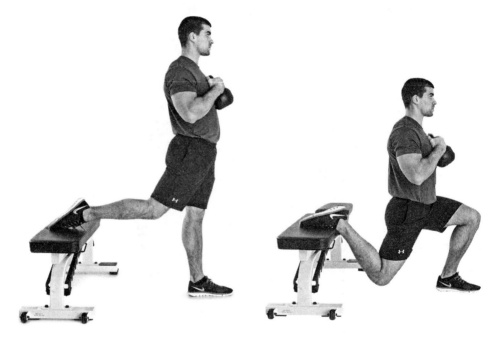

STEPUP

Assume the position: Grab a pair of dumbbells and stand facing a sturdy bench or step. If you have knee problems, I recommend a low step. No limitations? The higher the step, the harder your hip and thigh muscles will work. Place one foot on the step, with the other on the floor.

Work:

1. Push down through the heel of your working leg, and raise yourself up until your knee is straight and your nonworking foot reaches the step.

2. Without touching the step, lower your nonworking foot to the floor and begin the next rep. Don't push off the floor; the top leg does the work.

3. Finish the set, then switch legs and repeat.

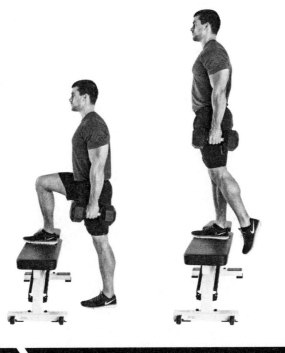

BIG-BOY TIP:

Every loading option noted for lunge variations can be used here.

▶ *Barbell, kettlebells, sandbag, weight plate*

▶ *Single or double dumbbells or kettlebells*

▶ *At your sides, at shoulder height, overhead, or in the rack position*

KETTLEBELL SWING

Assume the position: Set a kettlebell on the floor in front of you. Stand over it with your feet wide apart and angled out slightly. Push your hips back and grab it with both hands. Tighten everything.

Work:

1. Swing the weight back between your legs.

2. Snap your hips forward as you straighten your torso. This is a "Bam!" kind of movement. The weight should fly forward to about chest level. Don't deliberately lift it any higher than that.

3. Immediately pull it back down as you push back your hips for the next rep.

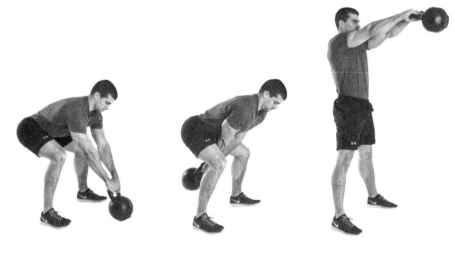

BIG-BOY TIP:

You can get really strong, really fast with swings. You can also hurt yourself if you don't approach them with the same caution as heavy deadlifts and squats. The deadlift is actually a good model for the loading stage of the exercise, when you're pulling the kettlebell back and setting your hips. As with the deadlift, you want to contract your lats, which pulls your shoulders down and fixes your lower back in a strong, safe position. Then, when you snap your hips forward, your glutes will both drive the movement and benefit most from it.

GLUTE BRIDGE

It's exactly like the warmup exercise shown in Chapter 10, except with a barbell across your pelvis. If you don't think the confluence of "barbell" and "pelvis" sounds promising—and why would you?—some precautions are in order.

A commercial gym will probably have foam pads that wrap around the barbell. They're designed to cushion the neck for back squats, which is why they're most often referred to as squat pads. I don't recommend them for that exercise; if the bar hurts your neck, there's a simple solution: Don't squat with the bar on your neck! It should sit on your traps, not your cervical spine. But the pad is perfect for glute bridges. If you train at home, you can buy a cheap one for $10 online, or spring for a $25 commercial-grade pad at performbetter.com and other sites. Or you can make your own out of foam padding or a couple towels.

Assume the position:

1. Load a barbell, and then wrap that rascal with something more groin-friendly than solid steel.

2. Sit on the floor facing it with your legs straight. Roll the bar over your feet and up to your lap, with the center of the bar on your body's midline.

3. Now lie on your back with your knees bent, and feet flat on the floor and a comfortable distance apart. Grab the bar with your hands about shoulder-width apart, and tighten everything up.

Work:

1. Push your hips straight up until your body forms a straight line from your chest to your knees.

2. Hold, feeling the squeeze in your glutes but not in your lower back.

3. Lower your hips to the floor and repeat.

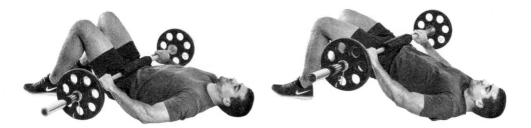

Carry

The carry is a simple exercise. You pick up the weights the same way you'd lift them for any other exercise—that is, *carefully*. Stand straight, striving for the same posture you'd have if you weren't holding something heavy. Now . . . walk. One foot in front of the other. The heavier the weights, the harder it is. There are four types of carries that should work well as part of the Lean Muscle Plan.

FARMER'S WALK

Hold a heavy thing in each hand. Dumbbells are the most convenient, but the bigger they are, the harder they are to walk with. Serious strength athletes use farmer's bars—barbells with a handle in the middle. (You can buy a pair for about $300.) Or you can use a hex bar.

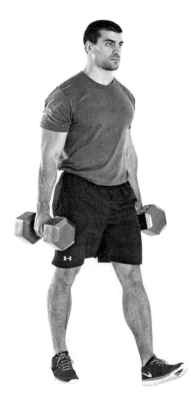

SUITCASE CARRY

Hold a heavy thing in one hand, and then walk as if the load is balanced. Obviously, you want to do the same number of steps with the weight to each side.

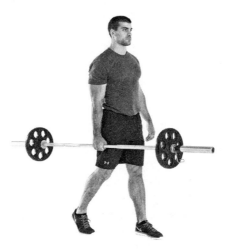

OVERHEAD CARRY

Hold anything you want overhead with straight arms: barbell, weight plate, sandbag, two dumbbells or kettlebells.

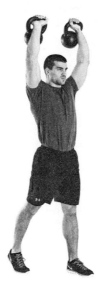

WAITER'S WALK

Hold one weight overhead or at shoulder height with a single arm. My favorite is the kettlebell bottoms-up carry: Grab the handle and hold the kettlebell upside-down in front of your shoulder. Lift your upper arm just enough to challenge your shoulder muscles. Stop walking when the weight slips or your shoulder can no longer hold the original position.

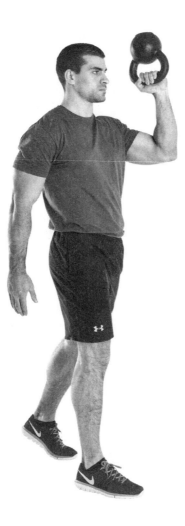

PUSHUP

Done right, the pushup is an outstanding total-body exercise. It not only hits the featured muscles—the chest, front delts, and triceps—it's also a decent core exercise, one that can be made even better as you introduce elements of instability (as shown on page 256). It's also versatile: You can do pushups with your feet elevated to put more emphasis on the top part of your chest, move your hands closer together to work your triceps harder, or combine the two.

Assume the position:

You know what to do: hands directly below your shoulders, feet hip-width apart, body in a straight line from neck to ankles. But here's a tip from a guy with a history of shoulder problems: Before you begin, spread your fingers and rotate your shoulders outward, as if you're trying to screw your hands into the floor. This should create a slightly more stable position for your shoulders.

Work:

1. Bend your elbows and lower your body *as a unit* toward the floor.

2. Stop when your chest is an inch from the floor, or your upper arms are parallel to the floor, whichever comes first. A longer range of motion can be problematic for taller, thinner guys, the ones with arms like a stork's legs. (I can say that because I was one of those guys until my early twenties.)

3. Push yourself back up to the starting position. *Be sure to complete each repetition,* going to full extension of your elbows and full flexion of your chest and shoulders. Most guys (again, including me) cut the movement short so we can knock out more reps. You'll get better results from fewer reps and a longer range of motion than you will from cranking them out like you're getting paid by the dozen.

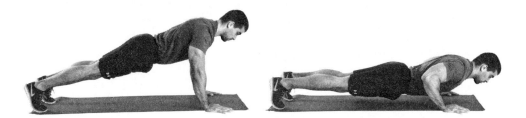

Any time it's easy to hit all the reps, make it harder. Some suggestions:

1. Elevate your feet.

2. Move your hands closer together, which puts more emphasis on your triceps.

3. Add a weight vest or another form of resistance. Don't do anything crazy, like having someone stack weight plates on your back, unless you have perfect confidence in your form. As future mothers will warn their children, just because you saw someone do it on YouTube doesn't mean it's a good idea.

4. Stagger your hands, so one is farther forward. Do 2 sets, each with a different arm forward. It's not only a unique challenge for your chest and shoulder muscles, it's a pretty good core workout as well.

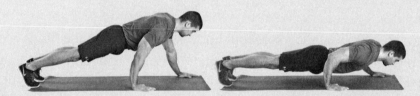

5. Put your hands on a pair of same-size medicine balls, or both hands on one ball. When Stuart McGill tested this move at his University of Waterloo lab, the abdominal muscles of his subjects were 75 percent active. That's one of the highest measurements I can recall from any study of core-muscle activation.

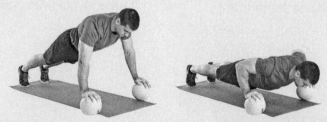

6. Create instability, either by putting your feet on a Swiss ball or in the loops of a suspension system, or by doing the same thing with your hands.

T PUSHUP

Assume the position:

Get into the basic pushup position.

Work:

1. Lower yourself to the floor, as in a standard pushup.

2. As you come up, rotate your body as you raise your right hand overhead. Follow your arm with your eyes. At the top, your arms should form a straight line perpendicular to the floor. Your head and torso will form the other part of the T.

3. Return to the starting position and immediately begin the next pushup.

4. As you come up, rotate the opposite direction as you raise your left arm.

5. Continue alternating. Each pushup counts as 1 repetition. So in a set of 12, for example, you'll do 6 to each side.

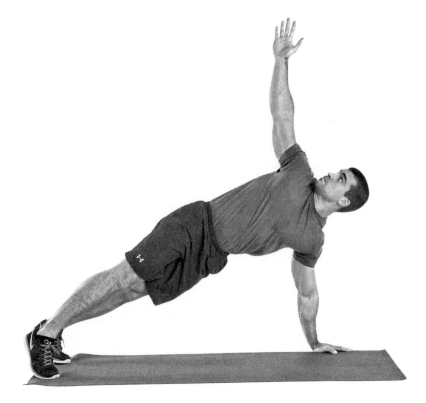

T pushups are prescribed in Phase One, Workout 3. Since you want to do max reps on each set, I recommend using just your body weight for the first workout. That gives you a baseline to build from. If you get 14 or more per set—that is, at least 7 to each side—add weight for your next workout. There are two ways to do it.

Single dumbbell: *Hold a dumbbell with one hand and do as many pushups as you can, all to the same side, lifting the weight from the floor to overhead. Switch the dumbbell to the other hand and do the same number of pushups.*

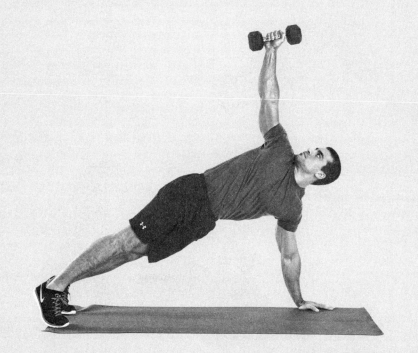

Two dumbbells: *Start with a dumbbell in each hand and alternate sides for each rep. This works best with hexagonal dumbbells. You can do it with round ones (I confess it's fun to try), but make sure you understand the risk.*

PIKE PUSHUP

This variation works your shoulders more than your chest, and it's a good complementary exercise on the days you do bench presses.

Assume the position:

Get into pushup position, only with your hips up in the air and flexed 90 degrees.

Work:

1. Lower your body toward the floor, keeping your hips bent at the same angle. Stop just short of hitting the floor with your face.

2. Push back up to the starting position.

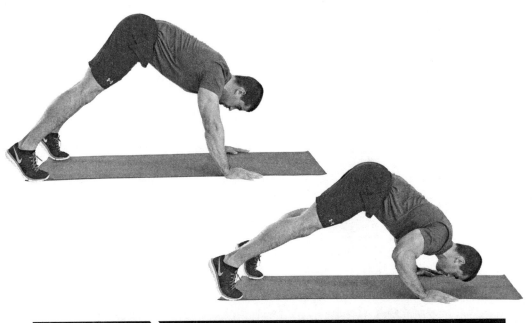

BIG-BOY TIP:

The inverted pushup—a pike pushup with your feet elevated—is one of my favorite exercises that I never used until recently. (I'm sure it's been around forever.) With your feet on a bench or box and your hips bent 90 degrees, you can get completely or nearly vertical. You can move your hands closer together to increase the range of motion and work your triceps a little harder. It's a great shoulder exercise either way.

CABLE ONE-ARM CHEST PRESS

Here's a *real* horizontal press, and also a magnificent core exercise. I'll describe it for a cable machine, but you can also use a resistance band.

Assume the position:

Attach a D-shaped handle to a cable pulley and set it to chest height. Grab the handle with both hands and pull it to your chest. Now, holding it with just your left hand, stand with your back to the weight stack and your legs in a split stance, with your right leg ahead of your left and your knees bent slightly. Tighten everything up.

Work:

1. Push the cable straight out from your shoulder.
2. Return to the starting position.
3. Do all your reps, switch sides, and repeat the set.

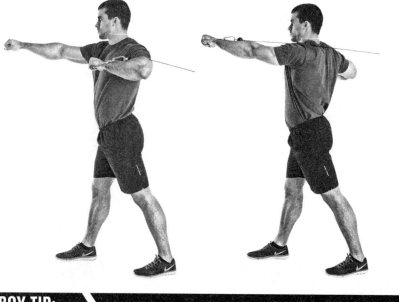

BIG-BOY TIP:

Keep your hips square throughout the full repetition, moving them as little as possible. You want your shoulders to rotate and your arm to extend, but everything else should stay firmly in place.

DUMBBELL OR KETTLEBELL SINGLE-ARM SHOULDER PRESS

Assume the position:

Grab a weight. If it's a dumbbell, hold it just above your shoulder, with your palm turned in. If it's a kettlebell, hold it in the rack position. Your hand will be at the top of your chest, while the bell will be wedged between your forearm and deltoid as shown. Take a wider stance than you would for the two-arm shoulder press, and hold your nonworking arm out to your side for balance.

Work:

1. With a dumbbell, press it straight up; with a kettlebell, the motion is more of a semicircle, since you're pressing out and up at the same time. You'll also probably lean a bit to your nonworking side for balance.

2. Lower the weight along the same trajectory.

3. Do all your reps, then switch sides and repeat.

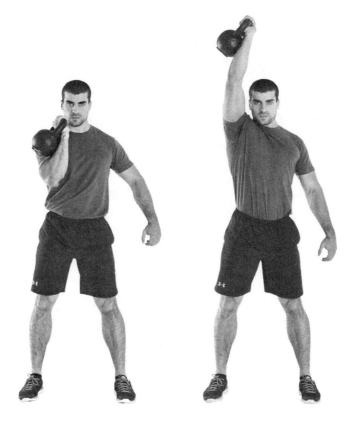

Cable Row Variations

You know, of course, that you have two pulling exercises per workout: one primary, one complementary or accessory. When possible, you want to use free weights or body weight on the first one. On the second I prefer to use a cable machine, so I wrote the programs that way.

Cables allow you to keep tension on your muscles throughout the movement, from a full stretch to a full contraction and back again. When you do those exercises on your feet or knees, you also have to brace your core. Do that with one arm at a time and you double the time your core is braced; do that for 10 or more reps to each side and you have a pretty awesome challenge to your core, back, and arms, and you might find yourself out of breath as well, making it the equivalent of interval training.

Here are your options.

ONE ARM OR TWO

For two-arm rows, any attachment you would use for lat pulldowns or arm exercises will work. That includes:

▶ Long bar, which allows a wide, overhand grip, good for hitting a range of upper-back muscles including lats, traps, and rear delts

▶ Angled bar, which allows several underhand grips, giving you more biceps work

▶ Triangle bar, which gives you a very close, neutral grip; that's a naturally strong position, allowing you to work with heavier weights

▶ Rope, which allows a slightly longer range of motion, since you don't have to stop when the bar hits your abdomen

▶ Two single handles, which, like the rope, allow a slightly increased range of motion; they also allow you to rotate from a neutral grip at the start to an underhand grip toward the end to hit your biceps more

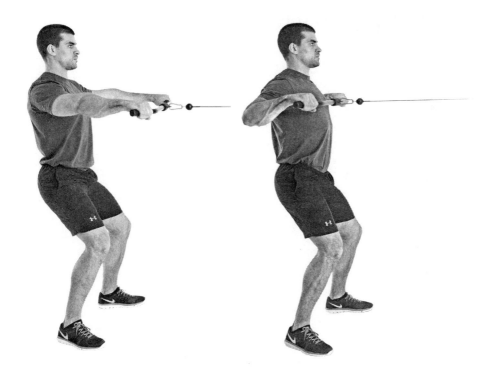

For one-arm rows, you really have just one good attachment option: the single handle. You can use a neutral or underhand grip, or start with the former and end with the latter. But that doesn't mean you can't switch up the exercise, as you'll see in the next section.

HIGH, LOW, OR ANYWHERE IN BETWEEN

A typical cable column at a commercial gym has up to 20 different pulley positions. Most of us, I suspect, use only two: the one at the top and the one at the bottom. In between you'll find a lot of new angles to work your back and arm muscles. Where you set the pulley will probably determine whether you use a. . .

PARALLEL OR SPLIT STANCE

When the pulley is at chest level or below, you'll probably want to stand with your feet parallel to each other, and your hips and shoulders square to the cable column. When the pulley is higher, you'll probably want to use a split stance, with one leg in front of the other. For one-arm rows, use the arm opposite the forward leg.

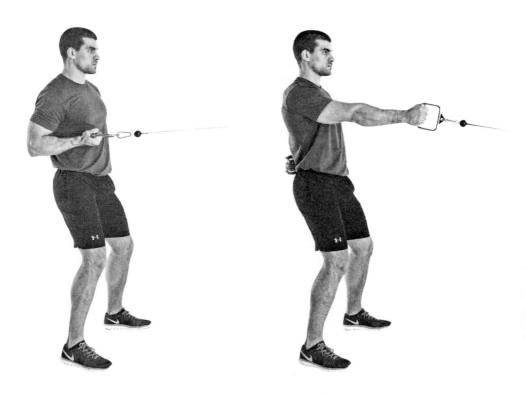

Biceps Curl Variations

When I see guys in the gym doing a lot of curls, they tend to be:

▶ Serious bodybuilders, who know exactly what they're doing

▶ Skinny kids, who entertain the magical idea that they can make their biceps grow out of proportion to all the larger muscles the biceps are designed to support

▶ Old guys who haven't trained in years, and have no idea what to do; rather than get help from a trainer, they'll sit on a bench and curl dumbbells for the next half-hour

There's no trick to curling a barbell or dumbbell: You stand holding the bar or dumbbells with straight arms. Then you bend your elbows and lift the weights up to the top of your chest. I doubt if there's much advantage to any particular curl over any other. The biceps are a simple muscle, originating in the shoulder and inserting into the elbow. They mainly do one thing: bend your elbow. Your goal is to get the most biceps development with the least time invested in specialized exercises and the lowest risk of injury.

Barbell curls, in theory, should be the go-to exercise, since they allow you to work with the heaviest weights. But they're really tough on your forearms.

Machine curls just seem like a terrible idea, since they force your shoulders, elbows, and wrists to conform to the machine's specifications.

Dumbbell curls make more sense, since your arms operate independently and accommodate your own biomechanical quirks.

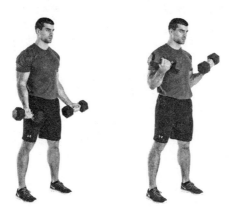

Cable curls are my favorite, since they're easiest on the joints and, like cable rows, allow continuous tension throughout the range of motion. You have all the same options I just described for cable rows—same attachments, hand positions, and pulley height.

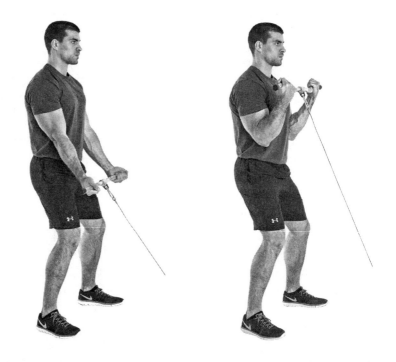

BIG-BOY TIPS: ▶

For maximum biceps development, use a range of reps and hand positions throughout the program.

▶ *Chinups for low reps (probably the best biceps exercise in the program)*

▶ *Lat pulldowns with a neutral grip for medium and/or high reps (great for forearm development and upper-arm thickness)*

▶ *Inverted rows with an overhand grip for medium reps*

▶ *Cable rows (single or double arm) for medium to high reps, using a variety of grips*

Triceps Exercises

The triceps straighten your elbow while it's bent but they also help pull your arms down to your sides when they're extended overhead or out in front of you. So they have a (very minor) role in exercises like pullups and lat pulldowns. You can take advantage by strategically expanding your range of motion on a couple of overhead exercises.

CABLE OVERHEAD TRICEPS EXTENSION

Use a high pulley with a rope or bar attachment. If you use a bar, you want an overhand grip that's just inside shoulder width. Stand with your back to the cable column and take a split stance, with your elbows bent and your upper arms slightly behind the plane of your torso (not shown here). Pull your upper arms forward as you straighten your elbows.

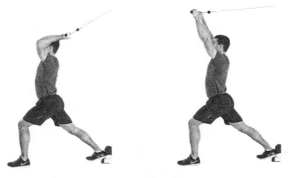

DUMBBELL PRONE TRICEPS EXTENSION

Grab two dumbbells and lie on your back on a flat bench. Start with your arms straight and angled back slightly—not perpendicular to the floor, in other words. Bend your elbows so the weights descend behind your head, then straighten them. You can also do this with an EZ-curl bar.

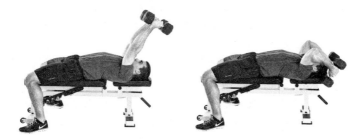

For triceps growth, it's hard to beat heavy presses. The dumbbell incline crush press, shown in the previous chapter, is probably the best triceps exercise in the program. To get maximum development, you can try some or all of these adjustments.

If you do barbell bench presses, *try a narrower grip (your thumbs 12 to 18 inches apart).*

If you do barbell shoulder presses, *add partial reps at the end of your final set.*

Pushups are easy to tweak: *If you have no shoulder problems, you can do diamond pushups, with your thumbs and forefingers touching.*

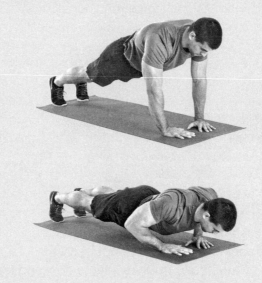

When you do overhead carries, *use a barbell, and carry it with your elbows bent slightly. This adds an isometric challenge for your triceps, and also seems to work the shoulders and upper traps a bit more (unless that's just my imagination).*

Then there's the most popular triceps exercise in the gym: the cable extension. *It's popular because it requires the least skill and hits the muscles as directly as possible. Everyone knows how to do it, and if you think it works for you, by all means include it in your program.*

EXERCISES YOU WON'T SEE IN THE LEAN MUSCLE PLAN

Parallel-Bar Dip

The goal: Build your chest, shoulders, and triceps

The problem: Any time you push a heavy weight with your arms behind your torso, you put your shoulders in a vulnerable position. Unless you're a gymnast, I don't think the risk is worth it.

Shrug

The goal: Build your upper trapezius

The problem: When you do the deadlifts, carries, and shoulder presses in this program with the heaviest weights you can manage for the specified sets and reps, you should build size and strength in your upper traps that's proportional to your overall development. The only way to create disproportionate upper traps is to use weights that are heavier than those you use for the other exercises. If you're doing it right, it should feel as if your upper torso is coming apart. That's a dangerous feeling, which is why you almost never see guys at your gym shrugging weights that are close to their max deadlift, much less beyond that max. I'm sure it makes sense to them, but it looks like a waste of time and energy to me.

Fly

The goal: Target chest muscles directly

The problem: Unless you're a serious bodybuilder, I see no good reason to do flies. The movement of your upper arms in a fly is exactly the same as in a bench press. Technically, they're both causing shoulder flexion. The only difference is that the elbows are open wider, putting the weights farther from the midline of your body. That stretch you feel is a sign of how big a risk you're taking with your shoulders.

SPECIAL TOPIC

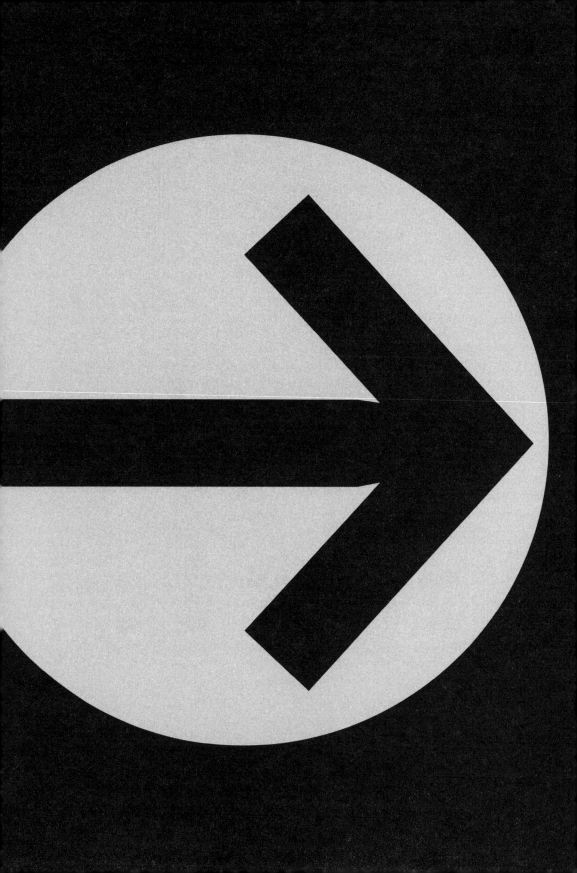

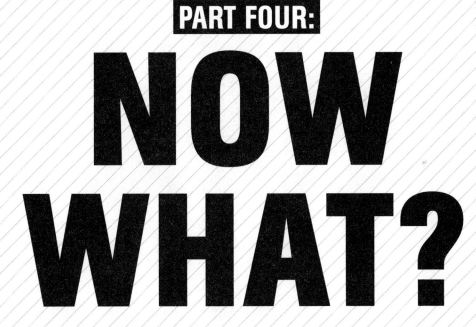

PART FOUR:
NOW WHAT?

CHAPTER 15

THE QUESTIONS WE KNOW YOU'LL ASK

What do I do if my target calories are different than the examples given in Chapter 8?

Pick the one that comes closest to your target body weight. Use that as an example of how to get the right amount of protein. Then adjust fat and carbs accordingly. It's easiest to do this as Alan does, with increments based on food types.

A cup of starches, for example, is around 200 calories. That's about the same whether it's pasta, rice, or beans. It's the equivalent of two slices of bread, or a couple small potatoes.

With fats, a tablespoon of nut butter is about 100 calories. One-third cup of nuts is about 200 calories.

These templates don't really match the way I think about food, or how I plan meals. What's up with that?

The templates show you one possible way to hit your calorie and macro-nutrient targets, while also getting a healthy mix of foods rich in vitamins and minerals. In Alan's experience, most of us do better when we stick to a template *at first*.

If your goal is to change your weight, and to maintain that new weight, no matter if it's lower or higher, you need knowledge and skills you don't currently have. Alan's templates are a great way to learn what the right amount of food for you looks like and feels like.

The goal isn't to measure every increment of food we eat from now until the day our robot overlords decide to pull the plug. It's to find the sweet spot, and then stay there. Once you have it, feel free to experiment and find something that better matches your preferences.

And if your experiments don't work? Go back to the template. It will always be there when you need it. Just remember you don't have to be a slave to it. (Unless the robots say you should.)

How long should I do the workouts?

As written, they would take an experienced lifter about 14 weeks to go from the first workout of Phase One to the end of Phase Three. But very few of us train that way. We get thrown off by work, vacations, weather, illness. Most of those breaks are unplanned, but in a way they're a blessing.

Let's say you're a lifter who's between beginner and intermediate status: You've been working out for several years, but you've rarely, if ever, done a progressive program with the goal of getting stronger each week. When you push yourself like that, you build up some residual fatigue.

Then one week your work piles up, or a freak snowstorm hits, or your company sends you out of town with a packed schedule and no chance to find a gym and train. You think you've blown it because you missed a couple workouts. But when you get back to the gym, you realize you're stronger, and you crush the workout with energy you haven't mustered in weeks. Those days off weren't wasted at all. Your body put them to good use.

It takes you 16 weeks to do a program that looks like 14 weeks on paper, but you actually accomplish more than you would if you blasted straight through without ever missing a workout.

Can I repeat the workouts?

Sure. In fact, if you've never done this type of program, you may actually get more out of it the second time. You'll be more skilled at the exercises that were new at the beginning, and you'll have a better idea of which options and variations work best in different parts of the program.

That second time through is especially useful if you're better at chinups or pullups than you were on the first go-round. It's a much more intense program with those exercises instead of lat pulldowns.

How do I get answers to all the other questions that will come up?

You can go to the forums at menshealth.com, or e-mail me via my Web site (louschuler.com), or find us on any of the usual social media outlets. We aren't shy, and we're happy to help if we can.

NOTES:

INTRODUCTION

World population: There's a nifty feature at Wikipedia (en.wikipedia.org/wiki/World_population) that updates this total frequently.

Metabolic homeostasis: Michael Rosenbaum and Rudolph Leibel, "Adaptive thermogenesis in humans," *International Journal of Obesity* (2010), 34: S47–S55 (hereafter cited as Rosenbaum and Leibel).

Weekends and holidays: Chad Cook et al, "Relation between holiday weight gain and total energy expenditure among 40- to 69-year-old men and women (OPEN study)," *American Journal of Clinical Nutrition* (2012), 95: 726–731.

Fitness event in Little Rock: The event is the Fitness Summit (thefitnesssummit.com), which was then called the JP Fitness Summit, after Jean-Paul Francoeur, who launched the event and hosted it at his gym the first 6 years. Starting in 2009, the Summit moved to Kansas City, Missouri, where it's hosted by Nick Bromberg. Both authors are heavily involved. Lou is the emcee and typically the first presenter; Alan, who has become the event's rock star, runs the anchor leg.

Boring nutrition experts: By the way, this doesn't apply to any of our friends. You guys are great. We're talking about the other ones. Admit it: You complain about them, too.

"Bonkers": If you're wondering how to distinguish a crackpot from a legit nutrition scientist, the "tell" is often the research used to back up his arguments. Generally speaking, the older the studies, the more batshit the idea. I'm not saying that research has an expiration date, but a solid premise can almost always be supported by research published in the past 3 to 5 years. A nutty premise is often supported by cherry-picked studies, willfully ignoring newer, better-designed research that contradicts a presenter's ideas.

Broscience: For a good explanation, do a Google search for "What Is Broscience? Deciphering Fact and Fiction in your Fitness Quest," by Brett Warren.

CHAPTER 1

Calories don't matter: Gary Taubes, "The science of obesity: what do we really know about what makes us fat?" *BMJ* (2013), 346:f1050.

Paleo diet: Debunking some of the odd claims made by paleo enthusiasts could be a full-time job. Several books published in the past few years are both good and corrective: *Paleofantasy: What Evolution Really Tells Us about Sex, Diet, and How We Live,* by Marlene Zuk (New York: W.W. Norton, 2013), specifically addresses the assertion that preagricultural humans were perfectly adapted to their environment. The environment changes, she argues, and humans have been especially good at changing along with it. It's an okay book, but it would have been better if it didn't at times read like an exercise in "nutpicking"—choosing the most outrageous statements on blogs and forums and responding to them as if they represent the entire group.

Much better is *The 10,000 Year Explosion: How Civilization Accelerated Human Evolution*, by Gregory Cochran and Henry Harpending (New York: Basic Books, 2009). The chapter on how lactose tolerance spread so quickly is by itself worth the price of the book.

"Get used to disappointment": One of many great lines from the movie *The Princess Bride*.

Single-set training to failure: This was originally promoted by Arthur Jones, who invented Nautilus machines and built the company that promoted the equipment, along with his unique ideas about how to use it effectively. It has adherents today, including a friend of mine, Ellington Darden, PhD, a former colleague of Jones's. I edited one of his books, *The New High-Intensity Training* (Emmaus, PA: Rodale, 2004).

CrossFit: For a good explanation of the potential dangers of CrossFit workouts, and the group's often casual disregard of them, see two articles at medium.com: "CrossFit's Dirty Little Secret," by Eric Robertson (September 25, 2013), and "Why I Quit CrossFit," by Jason Kessler (July 15, 2013).

Historic human proportions: This impression comes from many sources over the years. The most recent is *The Sports Gene: Inside the Science of Extraordinary Athletic Performance*, by David Epstein (New York: Current, 2013; hereafter cited as *The Sports Gene*). Although the entire book is terrific, I especially enjoyed the sections attempting to explain why so many athletes from small population groups rise to the top of different sports.

Muscle hypertrophy mechanisms: Brad Schoenfeld, "The mechanisms of muscle hypertrophy and their application to resistance training," *Journal of Strength and Conditioning Research* (2010), 24(10): 2857–2872.

Muscle damage vs. muscle soreness: Brad Schoenfeld and Bret Contreras, "Is postexercise muscle soreness a valid indicator of muscular adaptations?" *Strength and Conditioning Journal* (October 2013), 16–21.

Physical attractiveness: David A. Frederick and Martie G. Haselton, "Why is muscularity sexy? Tests of the fitness indicator hypothesis," *Personality and Social Psychology Bulletin* (2007), 33(8): 1167–1183.

Men's Health *article on golden ratio:* "The Perfect Body Formula," by John Barban, ran in the July 2008 issue on pages 138 to 140. You can check out an online version (www.menshealth.com/ fitness/muscle-building-strategy-v-shaped-torso), or view scans of the article as it appeared in the magazine by searching Google Books.

CHAPTER 2

Water in human body: John D. Kirschmann and Nutrition Search, Inc., *Nutrition Almanac*, 6th ed. (New York: McGraw-Hill, 2007), 85 (hereafter cited as *Nutrition Almanac*).

Thermic effect of food: Thomas Halton and Frank Hu, "The effects of high protein diets on thermogenesis, satiety, and weight loss: a critical review," *Journal of the American College of Nutrition* (2004), 23(5): 373–385; Eric Jéquier, "Pathways to obesity," *International Journal of Obesity* (2002), 26(S2): S12–S17.

Estimates for TEF are all over the board. For protein the range is 20 to 35 percent. For carbs it's 5 to 15 percent, and for fat it depends on the study: Some say it's less than the TEF for carbs, some say they're about the same.

Protein and weight loss: Stijn Soenen et al, "Relatively high-protein or 'low-carb' energy-restricted diets for body weight loss and body weight maintenance?" *Physiology & Behavior* (2012), 107(3): 374–380.

Diet quality: Ashima Kant, "Indexes of overall diet quality: a review," *Journal of the American Dietetic Association* (1996), 96(8): 785–791; Annika Wirt and Clare Collins, "Diet quality: what is it and does it matter?" *Public Health Nutrition* (2009), 12(12): 2473–2492; Patricia Waijers et al, "A critical review of predefined diet quality scores," *British Journal of Nutrition* (2007), 97(2): 219–231.

White bread: This is basic Wikipedia-level information.

Whey protein benefits: Gabriella Sousa et al, "Dietary whey protein lessens several risk factors for metabolic diseases: a review," *Lipids in Health and Disease* (2012), 11: 67.

Fruits and vegetables: Joel Kimmons et al, "Fruit and vegetable intake among adolescents and adults in the United States: percentage meeting individualized recommendations," *Medscape Journal* *of Medicine* (2009), 11(1): 26; Rui Liu, "Health benefits of fruits and vegetables are from additive and synergistic combinations of phytochemicals," *American Journal of Clinical Nutrition* (2003), 78(3): 517S–520S; Rui Liu, "Health-promoting components of fruits and vegetables in the diet," *Advances in Nutrition* (2013), 4(3): 384S–392S.

Data on the leading causes of death are from the National Center for Health Statistics (cdc.gov/nchs/fastats/lcod.htm).

Longevity champs: Clark-Knauss: "The Oldest Woman in the World Timeline," nealirc.org/gerontology/oldestwoman.html; Calment: Wikipedia; Sanchez-Blazquez: Associated Press, "World's Oldest Man, 112, Dies in NY," *New York Post*, September 15, 2013; Johnson: Associated Press, "Man Lived to 112 on Sausage-and-Waffles Diet," nbcnews.com, October 10, 2006.

What muscles are made of: Irwin Siegel, MD, *All about Muscle: A User's Guide* (New York: Demos, 2000), 28.

Protein requirements: Eric Helms et al, "A systematic review of dietary protein during caloric restrictions in resistance trained lean athletes: a case for higher intakes," *International Journal of Sports Nutrition and Exercise Metabolism* (epub ahead of print, 2013); Jacob and Gabriel Wilson, "Contemporary issues in protein requirements and consumption for resistance trained athletes," *Journal of the International Society of Sports Nutrition* (2006), 3: 7–27; Tyler Churchward-Venne et al, "Role of protein and amino acids in promoting lean mass accretion with resistance exercise and attenuating lean mass loss during energy deficit in humans," *Amino Acids* (2013), 45(2): 231–240; Stuart Phillips and Luc Van Loon, "Dietary protein for athletes: from requirements to optimum adaptation," *Journal of Sports Science* (2011), 29(S1): S29–S38 (hereafter cited as Phillips and Van Loon); Nancy Rodriguez et al, "Position Stand of the American Dietetic Association, Dietitians of Canada, and the American College of Sports Medicine: nutrition and athletic performance," *Journal of the American Dietetic Association* (2009), 109(3): 509–527; Bill Campbell et al, "International Society of Sports Nutrition position stand: protein and exercise," *Journal of the International Society of Sports Nutrition* (2007), 4: 8.

BCAA and leucine content: D. Joe Millward et al, "Protein quality assessment: impact of expanding our understanding of protein and amino acid needs for optimal health," *American Journal of Clinical Nutrition* (2008), 87(5): 1576S–1581S.

Making glucose from protein: Shane Bilsborough and Neil Mann, "A review of issues of dietary protein intake in humans," *International Journal of Sports Nutrition and Exercise Metabolism* (2006), 16(2): 129–152; Margriet Veldhorst et al, "Gluconeogenesis and energy expenditure after a high-protein, carbohydrate-free diet," *American Journal of Clinical Nutrition* (2009), 90(3): 519–526.

Carbs and sports: Richard Kreider et al, "ISSN exercise and sport nutrition review: research and recommendations," *Journal of the International Society of Sports Nutrition* (2010), 7: 7 (hereafter cited as Kreider et al); Adriano Lima-Silva et al, "Effects of a low- or high-carbohydrate diet on performance, energy system contribution, and metabolic responses during supramaximal exercise," *Applied Physiology, Nutrition, and Metabolism* (2013), 38(9): 928–934; Shaun Phillips et al, "Carbohydrate ingestion during team games exercise: current knowledge and areas for future investigation," *Sports Nutrition* (2011), 41(7): 559–585.

Average carb intake: Gregory Austin et al, "Trends in carbohydrate, fat, and protein intakes and association with energy intake in normal-weight, overweight, and obese individuals: 1971–2006," *American Journal of Clinical Nutrition* (2011), 93(4): 836–843.

Longest-lived people: Dan Buettner, *Blue Zones* (Washington, DC: National Geographic, 2008). In addition to the three groups mentioned, Buettner profiles people in Okinawa, where the plant-based diet includes both starchy carbs like rice and nonstarchy ones like soybeans; and Loma Linda, California, where the Seventh-Day Adventists he writes about avoid meat and eat lots of nuts and whole grains.

Alan and I have both used *Blue Zones* in articles and presentations as an easy way to refute militant paleo-diet advocates. If humans aren't supposed to eat grains or beans because they haven't been in the food chain long enough for our bodies to adapt to them, how come the longest-lived people in the world eat so many grains and beans?

Of course, our argument is somewhat facetious. It's silly to think you can live longer by adopting the diet of people who live a long time without also adopting their low-stress lifestyles, which include strong (and typically isolated) communities. All the Blue Zones are in temperate parts of the world where people spend a lot of time outdoors and get tons of exercise. You can't replicate that by eating beans instead of a steak.

Insulin sensitivity and weight loss: Marc-Andre Cornier et al, "Insulin sensitivity determines the effectiveness of dietary macronutrient composition on weight loss in obese women," *Obesity Research* (2005), 13(4): 703–709.

Carbohydrate recommendations: Kreider et al, 2010.

Fiber and disease prevention: Dagfinn Aune et al, "Dietary fiber, whole grains, and risk of colorectal cancer: systematic review and dose-response meta-analysis of prospective studies," *BMJ* (2011), 343: d6617; Robert Post et al, "Dietary fiber for the treatment of type 2 diabetes mellitus: a meta-analysis," *Journal of the American Board of Family Medicine* (2012), 25(1): 16–23; Seamus Whelton et al, "Effect of dietary fiber intake on blood pressure: a meta-analysis of randomized, controlled clinical trials," *Journal of Hypertension* (2005), 23(3): 475–481; Kya Grooms et al, "Dietary fiber intake and cardiometabolic risks among US adults, NHANES 1999-2010," *American Journal of Medicine* (2013), 126(12): 1059–1067; Bernard Venn and Jim Mann, "Cereal grains, legumes, and diabetes," *European Journal of Clinical Nutrition* (2004), 58(11): 1443–1461; Ingrid Flight and Peter Clifton, "Cereal grains and legumes in the prevention of coronary heart disease and stroke: a review of the literature," *European Journal of Clinical Nutrition* (2006), 60(10): 1145–1159.

Fiber and weight loss: Lorena Trigueros et al, "Food ingredients as anti-obesity agents: a review," *Critical Reviews in Food Science and Nutrition* (2013), 53(9): 929–942; Geoffrey Livesey, "Energy values of unavailable carbohydrate and diets: an inquiry and analysis," *American Journal of Clinical Nutrition* (1990), 51(4): 617–637; David Baer et al, "Dietary fiber decreases the metabolizable energy content and nutrient digestibility of mixed diets fed to humans," *Journal of Nutrition* (1997), 127(4): 579–586; Britt Burton-Freeman, "Dietary fiber and energy regulation," *Journal of Nutrition* (2000), 130(2): 272S–275S; Cheryl Rock, "Primary dietary prevention: is the fiber story over?" *Recent Results in Cancer Research* (2007), 174: 171–177.

Fiber guidelines: US Department of Agriculture, "Dietary Guidelines for Americans 2010," health. gov/dietaryguidelines/2010.asp.

Fiber content of foods (and other general fiber information): Linus Pauling Institute, lpi. oregonstate.edu/infocenter/phytochemicals/fiber.

History of low-fat diets: Ann La Berge, "How the ideology of low fat conquered America," *Journal of the History of Medicine* (2008), 63(2): 139–177.

Changes to American food supply: Lisa Harnack et al, "Temporal trends in energy intake in the United States: an ecologic perspective," *American Journal of Clinical Nutrition* (2000), 71(6): 1478–1484.

Human fat composition: Gray Malcom et al, "Fatty acid composition of adipose tissue in humans: differences between subcutaneous sites," *American Journal of Clinical Nutrition* (1989), 50(2): 288–291.

Daily PUFA consumption: Penny Kris-Etherton et al, "Polyunsaturated fatty acids in the food chain in the United States," *American Journal of Clinical Nutrition* (2000), 71(S): 179S–188S.

Benefits of omega-3 fatty acids: Julie Monaco et al, "Should you still recommend omega-3 supplements?" *Journal of Family Practice* (2013), 62(8): 422–424.

Ratio of omega-6 to omega-3 fatty acids: Artemis Simopoulos, "The importance of the ratio of omega-6/omega-3 essential fatty acids," *Biomedicine & Pharmacotherapy* (2002), 56(8): 365–379.

Health benefits of omega-6 fatty acids: Stephen Anton et al, "Differential effects of adulterated vs. unadulterated forms of linoleic acid on cardiovascular health," *Journal of Integrative Medicine* (2013), 11(1): 1–10.

Nuts: Emilio Ros, "Health benefits of nut consumption," *Nutrients* (2010), 2(7): 652–682; Vellingiri Vadivel et al, "Health benefits of nut consumption with special reference to weight control," *Nutrition* (2012), 28(11–12): 1089–1097; Michael Moss, "Are Nuts a Weight-Loss Aid?" *New York Times* (December 17, 2013).

History of hydrogenation: This is a grab bag from Wikipedia, crisco.com, and one of my books, *The New Rules of Lifting for Abs* (New York: Avery, 2010), pages 220 to 221. See also "The Battle Over Hydrogenation (1903–1920)," by Gary List and Michael A. Jackson (lipidlibrary.aocs.org/ history/hydrogenation/index.htm).

Saturated fat: Glen Lawrence, "Dietary fats and health: dietary recommendations in the context of scientific evidence," *Advances in Nutrition* (2013), 4(3): 294–302; Arne Astrup et al, "The role of reducing intakes of saturated fat in the prevention of cardiovascular disease: where does the evidence stand in 2010?" *American Journal of Clinical Nutrition* (2011), 93(4): 684–688; Melanie Warner, "A Lifelong Fight Against Trans Fats," *New York Times* (December 16, 2013).

Iron deficiency: "Iron and Iron Deficiency," cdc.gov/nutrition; "Micronutrient Deficiencies," who.int/nutrition; Cathy Fieseler, "Ironing Out the Details," *Running Times* (October/November 2013), 28–300.

Bodybuilders: Susan Kleiner et al, "Metabolic profiles, diet, and health practices of championship male and female bodybuilders," *Journal of the American Dietetic Association* (1990), 90(7): 962–967; Kleiner et al, "Nutritional status of nationally ranked elite bodybuilders," *International Journal of Sport Nutrition* (1994), 4(1): 54–69.

Popular diets: Jayson Calton, "Prevalence of micronutrient deficiency in popular diet plans," *Journal of the International Society of Sports Nutrition* (2010), 7: 24.

Obesity: Tania Markovic and Sharon Natoli, "Paradoxical nutritional deficiency in overweight and obesity: the importance of nutrient density," *Medical Journal of Australia* (2009), 190(3): 149–151.

Multivitamins: Dominik Alexander et al, "A systematic review of multivitamin-multimineral use and cardiovascular disease and cancer incidence and total mortality," *Journal of the American College of Nutrition* (2013), 32(5): 339–354.

Vitamin D: Robert Heaney, "Vitamin D: criteria for safety and efficacy," *Nutrition Reviews* (2008), 66 (S2): S178–S181.

Celiac disease and gluten intolerance: Alberto Rubio-Tapia et al, "The prevalence of celiac disease in the United States," *American Journal of Gastroenterology* (2012), 107(10): 1538–1544; Daniel DiGiacomo et al, "Prevalence of gluten-free diet adherence among individuals without celiac disease in the USA: results from the Continuous National Health and Nutrition Examination Survey 2009–2010," *Scandinavian Journal of Gastroenterology* (2013), 48(8): 921–925.

Diet success and adherence: Michael Dansinger et al, "Comparison of the Atkins, Ornish, Weight Watchers, and Zone diets for weight loss and heart disease risk reduction: a randomized trial," *Journal of the American Medical Association* (2005), 293(1): 43–53; Hongyu Wu et al, "Dietary interventions for weight loss and maintenance: preference or genetic personalization?" *Current Nutrition Reports* (2013), 2(4): 189–198.

Lactose intolerance: "Lactose Intolerance and Health," Agency for Healthcare Research and Quality Evidence Reports (February 2010). See also "Lactose Intolerance" at Genetics Home Reference, ghr.nlm.nih.gov/condition/lactose-intolerance.

CHAPTER 3

Interest in health, nutrition, and exercise: These things really do run in cycles, as explained in fascinating detail by Ruth Engs, EdD, a professor of applied health science at Indiana University, in *Clean Living Movements: American Cycles of Health Reform* (New York: Praeger Publishers, 2000). Immediately before any surge of interest in health and fitness, the country goes through a latency period. The overall cycle is typically 80 to 100 years long.

According to Engs, the latest cycle began around 1920. That's when the fervor for health reform peaked with the passage of the Eighteenth Amendment to the US Constitution, which prohibited alcohol. The amendment's unpopularity coincided with a drop in interest in healthy living that continued through the Roaring Twenties, the Depression, World War II, and the Baby Boom.

Resurgent interest in health took many forms: the "running boom" of the 1970s, anti-smoking and anti-drunk-driving activism, the popularity of alternative medicine and organic food. Engs predicted it would peter out by the mid-2000s, but in many ways the current clean-living movement is still going strong. Just to pick one example, as Alan and I were working on these chapters the US Food and Drug Administration moved toward banning all trans fats (artificial fats created from other fats to make them more stable in prepared foods).

That sort of legislation was unthinkable when I was growing up in the '60s, when the first warning labels on cigarette packs ("Caution: Cigarette smoking may be hazardous to your health") were considered intrusive.

Cigarette jingles and slogans: Off the top of my head, I remember these:

"You can take Salem out of the country, but! You can't take the country out of Salem."

LSMFT: Lucky Strike means fine tobacco.

"You've come a long way, baby" (Virginia Slims).

"Call for Philip Morris!"

"I'd rather fight than switch." (I had to Google to remember that this was Tareyton's slogan.)

"Winston tastes good like a cigarette should."

Charles Atlas: His Dynamic Tension program, a system of body-weight exercises interspersed with lifestyle tips, is still available online at charlesatlas.com. The idea that you could build a decent body without access to equipment remains appealing. Innovative trainers like our friend Bret Contreras, author of *Bodyweight Strength Training Anatomy* (Champaign, IL: Human Kinetics, 2013), offer high-quality programs for those times when you need to train but can't get to a gym.

Atlas himself seems to have been a true gentleman, but Dynamic Tension was always a marketing ploy. It was created by Frederick Tilney, a bodybuilder and marketing whiz who eventually worked with four of the most successful fitness entrepreneurs of the 20th century: Bernarr Macfadden (publisher of *Physical Culture* magazine), Bob Hoffman (founder of York Barbell and publisher of *Strength & Health*), Atlas, and Joe Weider (publisher of *Men's Fitness* and my employer from 1992 to 1997). Atlas himself was a well-known lifter and bodybuilder in the 1920s, and his rivals took umbrage with his claim that he built his famous physique with a handful of body-weight exercises.

In Joe Weider's autobiography, *Brothers of Iron* (Champaign, IL: Sports Publishing, 2006), he claims that Atlas once confronted him in a gym to explain why strength training was bad business. The margins, he explained, would never work. Inventory was expensive, and it cost too much to ship heavy things like barbell sets. Weider says Atlas offered the following advice: "Do what I do. Just run off sheets of paper and some pictures and charge the same amount of money."

I have no idea if this conversation occurred, or if it went the way Weider remembers. Weider possessed less humility or perspective about himself than anyone I've met, as I wrote in an article ("10 Most Influential Muscleheads," posted at t-nation.com on December 20, 2006) and in a review of *Brothers of Iron* for my blog ("Book of the Year," posted at louschuler.com on December 28, 2006). Which is a shame. I honestly think Weider, who died in early 2013, belongs in the pantheon of fitness visionaries, and should also be remembered as an important figure in publishing. His is also a terrific rags-to-riches story. Alas, it was hard to give him the credit he was due when he never passed up a chance to claim it for himself.

Termites: Tracy V. Wilson, "How Termites Work," howstuffworks.com (September 11, 2007).

Throwing and human evolution: Neil Roach et al, "Elastic energy storage in the shoulder and the evolution of high-speed throwing in *Homo*," *Nature* (2013), 498: 483–486. I relied on two news reports based on the study: "Pitch Perfect: Why Our Shoulders Are Key to Throwing," by Rhitu Chatterjee (npr.org, June 26, 2013), and "Throwing Is Key in Human Evolution, Study Suggests," by Fatimah Waseem (usatoday.com, June 27, 2013). An earlier article was also interesting and useful: "Armed and Deadly: Shoulder, Weapons Key to Hunt," by Christopher Joyce (npr.org, August 2, 2010).

Oldest spears: Arlette Kouwenhoven, "World's Oldest Spears," *Archaeology* (May/June 1997), 50(3); archive.archaeology.org.

Squat: Paul Comfort et al, "Are changes in maximal squat strength during preseason training reflected in changes in sprint performance in rugby league players?" *Journal of Strength and Conditioning Research* (2012), 26(3): 772–776.

Farmer's walk: Stuart McGill et al, "Comparison of strongman events: trunk muscle activation and lumbar spine motion, load, and stiffness," *Journal of Strength and Conditioning Research* (2009), 23(4): 1148–1161.

Core strength: Stuart McGill, *Ultimate Back Fitness and Performance* (Waterloo, ON: Wabuno Publishers, 2004), pages 80–81 (hereafter cited as *Ultimate Back Fitness*).

Can't isolate individual muscles: Eyal Lederman, "The myth of core stability," *Journal of Bodywork & Movement Therapies* (2010), 14: 84–98.

Muscle Beach: Harold Zinkin with Bonnie Hearn, *Remembering Muscle Beach* (Santa Monica, CA: Angel City Press, 1999). He mentions his Universal machine just once, in the book's introduction.

The rest of the book is about Muscle Beach itself, with lots of warmly remembered stories about his fellow lifters and acrobats.

"Like something out of Star Trek": I don't know that my brother or I ever watched the original series during its initial run on network TV, which ended in 1969. But *Star Trek* was already in syndication by 1970 or '71, so I can justify using it as a point of reference.

Gold's Gym: Paul Solotaroff, "The Dawn of Bodybuilding," *Men's Journal* (February 2012). Solotaroff's article has a great anecdote about the original Gold's Gym in Venice, California. The first time future bodybuilding champion Robbie Robinson walked into the gym to train, he was confronted by Ken Waller, a former Mr. Universe and the gym's manager. Waller told Robinson that if he wanted to train there, he'd have to do 10 bench-press reps with 150-pound dumbbells. That's 300 total pounds. After Robinson gutted out the reps, Waller welcomed him to the club, which included Arnold Schwarzenegger and Franco Columbu, among other present and future stars. Then he ordered him to deadlift 700 pounds. What I love about the story—assuming it's truth-adjacent, if not 100 percent accurate—is that it shows how strong those golden-age bodybuilders were, and how much they valued strength.

CHAPTER 4

BMI: You can calculate your own BMI at nhlbi.nih.gov/guidelines/obesity/BMI/bmicalc.htm.

Twins and BMI: Nancy Segal et al, "Genetic and environmental contributions to body mass index: comparative analysis of monozygotic twins, dizygotic twins and same-age unrelated siblings," *International Journal of Obesity* (2009), 33(1): 37–41. The age range used in the study was enormous: The youngest were just under 4 years old, and the oldest were just over 55.

Height: *The Sports Gene*, 135.

Paul Anderson, and other naturals: Most of the stories of Anderson's strength come from single sources. One guy says he saw him do this; another guy says he saw him do that. But there are so many stories, told by serious strength athletes who had no reason to make them up, that you have to assume they're at least mostly true. I used two roundups here: "Paul Anderson, King of the Squat," by Clarence Bass (cbass.com, 1999), and "American Strength Legends: Paul Anderson" (samson-power.com, 1998).

I also used "The Truth about Bodybuilding Genetics," by Bret Contreras (t-nation.com, January 11, 2011), as well as an interview with record-setting powerlifter Andy Bolton at seriouspowerlifting.com. In that interview, Bolton claims to have squatted 220 kilograms—485 pounds—the first time he tried it. And not just that: He did 22 reps. His first deadlift, he says, was 260 kilograms, or 573 pounds. (His first bench press was a relatively modest 80 kilograms/176 pounds.)

A story like this seems impossible, even if you know Bolton went on to become the first to deadlift 1,000 pounds in a sanctioned meet, or that his best squat was a world-record 1,213 pounds. But if anybody could, the smart money would be on someone like Bolton, who won his first powerlifting meet at 21, just 3 years after he started lifting and 1 year after he started training for the sport.

You can find more stories, and better stories, about athletic prodigies throughout *The Sports Gene*.

Bone and muscle mass: *The Sports Gene*, 124.

Satellite cells and muscle growth: John Petrella et al, "Potent myofiber hypertrophy during resistance training in humans is associated with satellite cell-mediated myonuclear addition: a cluster analysis," *Journal of Applied Physiology* (2008), 104(6): 1736–1742.

The Sports Gene (pages 106 to 107) and "The Truth about Bodybuilding Genetics" also covered this research.

Endurance and athleticism: *The Sports Gene*, chapter 5.

Genetics and body fat: I could list a bunch of studies here, but the honest truth is that they would mostly be the same ones Bret used in "The Truth about Bodybuilding Genetics."

NBA demographics: Seth Stephens-Davidowitz, "In the NBA, Zip Code Matters," *New York Times* (November 2, 2013).

Gains for elite weightlifters: Steven Fleck and William Kraemer, *Designing Resistance Training Programs*, 3rd ed. (Champaign, IL: Human Kinetics, 2004), 14.

Adaptive thermogenesis: Rosenbaum and Leibel, 2010.

The quote is from César Boguszewski et al, "Neuroendocrine body weight regulation: integration between fat tissue, gastrointestinal tract, and the brain," *Endokrynologia Polska* (2010), 61(2): 194–206. I don't pretend to keep Polish medical journals at my bedside, but Alan apparently does. Or at least he downloads and cites them in *Alan Aragon's Research Review* (alanaragon. com/researchreview). He quoted the study in the final installment of a three-part series called "Clearing Up Common Misunderstandings that Plague the Calorie Debate," the lead article in his September 2013 issue. He also discussed adaptive thermogenesis in fascinating detail in part one of the series, in July 2013.

Exercise and weight loss: Pierpaulo De Feo, "Is high-intensity exercise better than moderate-intensity exercise for weight loss?" *Nutrition, Metabolism, and Cardiovascular Diseases* (2013), epub ahead of print.

Abs are made in the kitchen: I've pushed back against this one multiple times over the years. I made what I think is my strongest pro-exercise argument in "Smash Fat Faster" (*Men's Health*, November 2013, pages 146 to 149), which is one of my favorite magazine articles of the past few years. It presents some speculative but intriguing arguments on why people who do more vigorous exercise have more muscle and less fat, despite the fact they often eat more than people who have a higher body-fat percentage.

Another is a blog post: "Nutrition: What Do We Know, and How Do We Know It?" (louschuler.com, March 14, 2011).

Dave Draper quote: "Learn from My Mistakes: An Interview with Dave Draper," wannabebig.com (December 16, 2003).

Winners do quit: Seth Godin, *The Dip: A Little Book that Teaches You When to Quit (and When to Stick)* (New York: Portfolio, 2007), 31.

Fit the exercise to you: Nick Tumminello, "Deadlifts: One of the Most Functional Exercises for Everything," nicktumminello.com (November 6, 2013).

CHAPTER 5

NEAT study: James Levine et al, "Role of nonexercise activity thermogenesis in resistance to fat gain in humans," *Science* (1999), 283(5399): 212–214.

Rapid weight loss: Wim Saris, "Very-low-calorie diets and sustained weight loss," *Obesity Research* (2001), 9(S4): 295S–301S; James Anderson et al, "Long-term weight-loss maintenance: a meta-analysis of US studies," *American Journal of Clinical Nutrition* (2001), 74(5): 579–584; Lisa Nackers et al, "The association between rate of initial weight loss and long-term success in obesity treatment: does slow and steady win the race?" *International Journal of Behavioral Medicine* (2010), 17(3): 161–167; Ina Garthe et al, "Effect of two different weight-loss rates on body composition and strength and power-related performance in elite athletes," *International Journal of Sport Nutrition and Exercise Metabolism* (2011), 21(2): 97–104.

Moderate weight loss benefits: Rena Wing et al, "Benefits of modest weight loss in improving cardiovascular risk factors in overweight and obese individuals with type 2 diabetes," *Diabetes Care* (2011) 34(7): 1481–1486; George Blackburn, "Effect of degree of weight loss on health benefits," *Obesity Research* (1995), 3(S2): 211S–216S.

Healthy body-fat range: Ursula Kyle et al, "Body composition interpretation: contributions of the fat-free-mass index and the body-fat-mass index," *Nutrition* (2003), 19(7–8): 597–604; R. Paul Abernathy and David Black, "Healthy body weights: an alternative perspective," *American Journal of Clinical Nutrition* (1996), 63(S3): 448S–451S.

Athletes and body fat: Steven Fleck, "Body composition of elite American athletes," *American Journal of Sports Medicine* (1983), 11(6): 398–403; Lindy Rossow et al, "Natural bodybuilding competition preparation and recovery: a 12-month case study," *International Journal of Sports Physiology and Performance* (2013), 8: 582–592; Robert Withers et al, "Body composition changes in elite male bodybuilders during preparation for competition," *Australian Journal of Science and Medicine in Sport* (1997), 29(1): 11–16.

Body-fat classifications: These are just estimates, and aren't meant to correlate directly with body-mass index. An athlete with a BMI over 30 would be obese on that scale, but if he has less than 13 percent body fat, he'd be considered "lean" for our purposes. Conversely, a skinny-fat guy starting our program could be normal weight, or just slightly overweight, according to BMI, but still have a body-fat percentage north of 25 percent, putting him into our obese category.

Interestingly, some researchers have attempted to use body-fat percentage in the same way BMI is used: to make a judgment call about someone's health status based on their girth. But according to this editorial, there's no reliable association between body-fat percentage and risk of heart failure: Lan Ho-Pham et al, "More on body fat cutoff points," *Mayo Clinic Proceedings* (2011), 86(6): 584.

CHAPTER 6

Nutrition databases: Alan mostly used nutritiondata.com and the USDA Nutrient Database (ndb. nal.usda.gov/ndb/search/list). When those databases didn't have a particular detail he needed (like the fiber content of some of the more obscure or exotic foods), Google searches led him to caloriecount.about.com and fatsecret.com. I added a couple of data points from the previously cited *Nutrition Almanac*.

Dairy benefits: Beth Rice et al, "Meeting and exceeding dairy recommendations: effects of dairy consumption on nutrient intakes and risk of chronic disease," *Nutrition Reviews* (2013), 71(4); 209–223. While this review was written by dairy-industry scientists, the information comes from more than 50 studies.

CHAPTER 7

Meal frequency: Moira Taylor and John Garrow, "Compared with nibbling, neither gorging or a morning fast affect short-term energy balance in obese patients in a chamber calorimeter," *International Journal of Obesity and Related Metabolic Disorders* (2001), 25(4): 519–528; Wilhelmine Verboeket-van de Venne and K. Roel Westerterp, "Influence of the feeding frequency on nutrient utilization in man: consequences for energy metabolism," *European Journal of Clinical Nutrition* (1991), 45(3): 161–169; Marjet Munsters and Wim Saris, "Effects of meal frequency on metabolic profiles and substrate partitioning in lean healthy males," *PLoS One* (2012), 7(6): e38632; Hamid Farshchi et al, "Regular meal frequency creates more appropriate insulin sensitivity and lipid profiles compared with irregular meal frequency in healthy lean women," *European Journal of Clinical Nutrition* (2004), 58(7): 1071–1077.

Protein frequency: José Areta et al, "Timing and distribution of protein ingestion during prolonged recovery from resistance exercise alters myofibrillar protein synthesis," *Journal of Physiology* (2013), 591(9): 2319–2331.

Leucine: Phillips and Van Loon; Bart Pennings et al, "Amino acid absorption and subsequent muscle protein accretion following graded intakes of whey protein in elderly men," *American Journal of Physiology: Endocrinology and Metabolism* (2012), 302(8): E992–E999.

Long-term meal frequency: Paul Arciero et al, "Increased protein intake and meal frequency reduces abdominal fat during energy balance and energy deficit," *Obesity* (2013), 21: 1357–1366.

Breakfast: Priya Deshmukh-Taskar et al, "The relationship of breakfast skipping and type of breakfast consumed with overweight/obesity, abdominal obesity, other cardiometabolic risk factors and the metabolic syndrome in young adults. The National Health and Nutrition Examination Survey (NHANES): 1999–2006," *Public Health Nutrition* (2013), 16(11): 2073–2082; Andrew Brown et al, "Belief beyond the evidence: using the proposed effect of breakfast on obesity to show two practices that distort scientific evidence," *American Journal of Clinical Nutrition* (2013), 98(5): 1298–1308.

Protein timing: John Ivy and Robert Portman, *Nutrient Timing: The Future of Sports Nutrition* (Laguna Beach, CA: Basic Health, 2004), 8; Alan Aragon and Brad Schoenfeld, "Nutrient timing revisited: is there a post-exercise anabolic window?" *Journal of the International Society of Sports Nutrition* (2013), 10: 5.

Potential vitamin and mineral deficiencies: Micronutrient Information Center, Linus Pauling Institute at Oregon State University (lpi.oregonstate.edu/infocenter/multivitamin-mineral.html).

Fish-oil benefits: See examine.com/supplements/fish+oil for a complete rundown of every possible benefit that's been studied. (It's a *long* list.)

Fish oil and muscle hypertrophy: Gordon Smith et al, "Omega-3 polyunsaturated fatty acids augment the muscle protein anabolic response to hyperaminoacidemia-hyperinsulinemia in healthy young and middle-aged men and women," *Clinical Science* (2011), 121(6): 267–278.

Dueling fish-oil reviews: Sang Kwak et al, "Efficacy of omega-3 fatty acid supplements in the secondary prevention of cardiovascular disease," *JAMA Internal Medicine* (2012), 172(9): 686–694;

Javier Delgado-Lista et al, "Long-chain omega-3 fatty acids and cardiovascular disease: a systematic review," *British Journal of Nutrition* (2012), 107(S2): S201–S213; William Harris et al, "Omega-3 fatty acids and cardiovascular disease: new developments and applications," *Postgraduate Medicine* (2013), 125(6): 100–113.

Vitamin D: Kimberly Forrest and Wendy Stuhldreher, "Prevalence and correlates of vitamin D deficiency in the US," *Nutrition Research* (2011), 31(1): 48–54; Ian Berry and Kelsey Gee, "America's Milk Business in a 'Crisis,'" *Wall Street Journal* (December 11, 2012); Ian Reid et al, "Effects of vitamin D supplements on bone mineral density: a systematic review and meta-analysis," *The Lancet* (2014), 383(9912): 146–155; Philippe Autier et al, "Vitamin D status and ill health: a systematic review," *The Lancet Diabetes & Endocrinology* (2014), 2(1): 76–89; Tyler Barker et al, "Supplemental vitamin D enhances the recovery in peak isometric force shortly after intense exercise," *Nutrition & Metabolism* (2013), 10(1): 69; Stefan Pilz et al, "Effect of vitamin D supplementation on testosterone levels in men," *Hormone and Metabolism Research* (2011), 43(3): 223–225.

Magnesium: Andrea Rosanoff et al, "Suboptimal magnesium status in the United States: are the health consequences underestimated?" *Nutrition Reviews* (2012), 70(3); 153–164; *Nutrition Almanac.*

Weight-loss supplements: Melinda Manore, "Dietary supplements for improving body composition and reducing body weight: where is the evidence?" *International Journal of Sports Nutrition and Exercise Metabolism* (2012), 22(2): 139–154.

Muscle-building supplements: Jay Hoffman and Michael Falvo, "Protein: which is best?" *Journal of Sports Science and Medicine* (2004), 3: 118–130; Kreider et al; Thomas Buford et al, "International Society of Sports Nutrition position stand: creatine supplementation and exercise," *Journal of the International Society of Sports Nutrition* (2007), 4: 6.

Primates and alcohol: John Williams, "How to Eat Like a Caveman (the Real Kind)," louschuler.com, (November 6, 2013), louschuler.com/blog/how-to-eat-like-a-caveman-the-real-kind.

Alcohol and weight: Dominik Pesta et al, "The effects of caffeine, nicotine, ethanol, and tetrahydrocannabinol on exercise performance," *Nutrition & Metabolism* (2013), 10: 71.

CHAPTER 9

Training vs. working out vs. exercise: I first explained the distinctions I make when I use these terms in *The New Rules of Lifting for Life* (New York: Avery, 2012), on page 5, and reiterated them in *The New Rules of Lifting Supercharged* (New York: Avery, 2013), on page 16. I figured other fitness writers have come up with more or less the same ideas, although no specific one came to mind at the time I wrote those passages.

However, after writing this chapter, I saw nearly identical definitions of training and working out in "CrossFit: The Good, Bad, and the Ugly" by Mark Rippetoe (t-nation.com, December 2, 2013). Here's how Rip phrased it: "Exercise is physical activity for its own sake, a workout done for the effect it produces today, during the workout or right after you're through. Training is physical activity done with a longer-term goal in mind, the constituent workouts of which are specifically designed to reach that goal."

"A workout is only as good as the adaptations it produces": Lou Schuler and Alwyn Cosgrove, *The New Rules of Lifting* (New York: Avery, 2006), 34. This was New Rule #8. I apologize for quoting myself.

Adrenaline and fat loss: Hassane Zouhal et al, "Catecholamines and obesity: effects of exercise and training," *Sports Medicine* (2013), 43(7): 591–600.

John Wooden quote: I've also seen a shorter version of it: "The main ingredient of stardom is the team." Either way, I think his point is the one I'm trying to make.

Exercise order: Roberto Simão et al, "Influence of exercise order on the number of repetitions performed and perceived exertion during resistance exercises," *Journal of Strength and Conditioning Research* (2005), 19(1): 152–156.

There's quite a bit of research, a lot of it from this team at Gama Filho University in Brazil, showing that the order in which you do exercises in your workout helps determine the results. They test a series of exercises in both directions: One group starts with big-muscle exercises like bench presses and lat pulldowns, while another starts with biceps curls and triceps exercises. This one showed that you do the fewest reps on the final exercise in a workout, no matter which exercise it is. Their conclusions are consistent: whatever matters most, do first.

The golf-cart incident: I wrote about my daughter's injury in a blog post called "Things Break" (louschuler.com, August 8, 2009).

Weight-room injuries: Zachary Kerr et al, "Epidemiology of weight training-related injuries presenting to United States emergency departments, 1990 to 2007," *American Journal of Sports Medicine* (2010), 38(4): 765–771; Gregory Myer et al, "Youth versus adult 'weightlifting' injuries presenting to United States emergency rooms: accidental versus nonaccidental injury mechanisms," *Journal of Strength and Conditioning Research* (2009), 23(7): 2054–2060; Nicholas Bakalar, "Weight-Lifting Injuries on the Rise," *New York Times* (June 21, 2010).

CHAPTER 10

Hip abduction strength: Chad Waterbury, "Glute Training Science at MPI," chadwaterbury.com (November 26, 2013). Chad's blog post includes several more advanced exercises to build abduction strength. "MPI" refers to the Movement Performance Institute at USC, where Chad is currently studying to become a doctor of physical therapy.

CHAPTER 11

Situps and back health: Stuart McGill, *Low Back Disorders* (Champaign, IL: Human Kinetics, 2002), 105 (hereafter cited as *Low Back Disorders*).

Nick Tumminello: Nick is a longtime colleague and friend. The information he shared with me is derived from Core Training: Facts, Fallacies, and Top Techniques, a three-DVD set available from nicktumminello.com.

Dynamic neuromuscular stimulation: Clare Frank et al, "Dynamic neuromuscular stabilization and sports rehabilitation," *The International Journal of Sports Physical Therapy* (2013), 8(1): 62–73; Chad Waterbury, "A Uniquely Effective Core Exercise," chadwaterbury.com (June 13, 2013).

Dead bug sequence: These exercises come from Dean Somerset, Chad Waterbury, and Mike Robertson. (If I've borrowed from anyone else and forgotten to give him or her credit, I apologize.) The name "resurrected dead bug" comes from strength coach Dan John (more on Dan in the notes for Chapter 13).

Dead bug muscle activation: James Youdas et al, "An electromyographic analysis of the ab-slide exercise, abdominal crunch, supine double-leg thrust, and side bridge in healthy young adults: implications for rehabilitation professionals," *Journal of Strength and Conditioning Research* (2008), 22(6): 1939–1946. The supine double-leg thrust is the closest approximation I could find to the dead bug. The starting position is the same, but instead of one leg extending, both legs go out. The study showed extremely high muscle activation of all four muscles tested: rectus abdominis, external and internal obliques, and hip flexors.

Lumbar spine rotation range: *Low Back Disorders*, 88.

Pallof press: John Pallof is a physical therapist based in Worcester, Massachusetts. The exercise named was first popularized by Boston-area trainers Mike Boyle, Eric Cressey, and Tony Gentilcore. Variations described in Chapter 11 come from Nick Tumminello and Mike Robertson.

Muscle activation in rollout and jackknife: Rafael Escamilla et al, "Core muscle activation during Swiss ball and traditional abdominal exercises," *Journal of Orthopedic & Sports Physical Therapy* (2010), 40(5): 265–276 (hereafter cited as Escamilla et al, "Core muscle activation").

McGill curlup: *Ultimate Back Fitness*, 267–278.

Turkish getup origins: I tried and failed to find any authentic history of the exercise. But the combination of limited curiosity and mediocre search skills prevented me from getting beyond blog posts and online articles making unsupported assertions. Some of them seemed authoritative, but without citations, who knows?

CHAPTER 13

Benefits and risks of squats: Dan John, "Goblet Squats 101," t-nation.com (March 3, 2011). This article explains the accidental origin of the goblet squat, which turned out to be a superior way to teach athletes of all shapes, sizes, and abilities the basic mechanics of a fundamental movement pattern.

Deadlifts: Michael Boyle, "Lifts I Never Did, Used to Do, or Just Started Doing Again," t-nation.com (February 3, 2009). I edited this article; Mike was one of my favorite writers.

Sumo vs. conventional deadlifts: Rafael Escamilla et al, "A three-dimensional biomechanical analysis of sumo and conventional style deadlifts," *Medicine & Science in Sports & Exercise* (2000), 32(7): 1265–1275; Chris Beardsley, "How Do Conventional and Sumo Deadlifts Differ?" strengthandconditioningresearch.com (November 26, 2012).

Deadlift eye gaze: Mark Rippetoe, *Starting Strength*, 3rd ed. (Wichita Falls, TX: Aasgaard, 2011), 136–137.

Trap-bar deadlift: Chris Beardsley, "How Do Standard and Hex-Bar Deadlifts Differ?" strengthandconditioningresearch.com (December 10, 2012), strengthandconditioningresearch.com/2012/12/10/hex-bar-deadlifts; Paul Swinton et al, "A biomechanical analysis of straight and hexagonal barbell deadlifts using submaximal loads," *Journal of Strength and Conditioning Research* (2011), 25(7): 2000–2009; Jason Ferruggia, "Are Trap-Bar Deadlifts Safer than Straight-Bar Deadlifts?" jasonferruggia.com (July 11, 2011).

Barbell overhead press: John Fair, "The tragic history of the military press in Olympic and world championships competition, 1928–1972," *Journal of Sport History* (2001) 28(3): 345–374; Chris Colucci, "The Overhead Press: Bodybuilding's Forgotten Muscle Builder," t-nation.com (June 30, 2009).

CHAPTER 14

Pushup as core exercise: Escamilla et al, "Core muscle activation."

Pushup with hands on medicine balls: *Ultimate Back Fitness*, 287.

INDEX:

Boldface page references indicate illustrations. Underscored references indicate tables.

Fat, body
borderline obese case study (skinny-fat Stan), 92–93, 142–44
burning for energy (lipolysis), 72
energy movement in and out of, 25
estimating yours, 86–87
evolutionary adaptation and, 8
genetic determinants of, 66–68
healthiest range for, 85
obese case study (deskbound Dan), 91–92, 140–42
obesity, 24, 62
overweight, 24, 62
overweight case study (brotacular Bob), 94, 144–46
percentages for college athletes, 85–86, 85
percentages for six-pack abs, 86
percent of carbs in diet and, 24
protection against losing too much, 72
skinny-fat rubric, 69
target percentage, 87
underweight case study (bulking Barry), 95, 147–49
warmup routine and burning of, 155
Fat, dietary, 29–34
amount per day, 34
animal protein, high fat, 105
animal protein, lean to moderate fat, 104–5
animal protein, very lean, 101–3
brotacular Bob case study, 94
bulking Barry case study, 95
calories from, for target body weight, 90, 273
deskbound Dan case study, 91
fish oil supplements, 128–29, 138
heart disease risk and, 30, 33
low-fat diets, 4, 7, 26, 29–31
in meal plans, 137–38
in meat food group, 100
monounsaturated fatty acids (MUFAs), 31, 109–11
percent of calories from, 34
polyunsaturated fatty acids (PUFAs), 31–33, 111–12
saturated fats, 33–34, 109
skinny-fat Stan case study, 93
thermic effect of food for, 14
trans fats, 33

unsaturated fats, 31–33, 109–12
vegetable protein, high fat, 107–8
vegetable protein, lean to moderate fat, 107
vegetable protein, very lean, 106–7
Fat burning, 72, 155. See also Metabolism
Fat-rich foods
animal protein, very lean, 101–3
categories for, 108
crossover with other food groups, 100
food group for, 37
highest in monounsaturated fat, 109–11
highest in polyunsaturated fat, 111–12
highest in saturated fat, 109
mix of fatty acids in, 108
vegetable protein, high fat, 107–8
Fiber
amount needed, 28
benefits of, 27–28
food sources of, 28–29
"negative" calories with, 27–28
soluble vs. insoluble, 27
from supplements vs. foods, 28
in vegetables, 7
Fibrous vegetables, 37, 112–15
Fish oil supplements, 128–29, 138
Fluid, 138
Fly exercise, 269
Food Allergen Labeling and Consumer Protection Act, 41
Food allergies, 41–42
Food groups. See also Food lists; specific groups
crossover among, 99
in Lean Muscle Diet, 37, 99
mnemonic device for, 37, 99
rule of two for, 138
Food lists
animal protein, high fat, 105
animal protein, lean to moderate fat, 104–5
animal protein, very lean, 101–3
fibrous vegetables, 112–15
fruits, 120–21
grains and grain products, 116–17
highest in monounsaturated fat, 109–11
highest in polyunsaturated fat, 111–12
highest in saturated fat, 109
milk and dairy products, 119–20
numbers rounded in, 99–100